IMPLEMENTATION AND MONITOR... ...G

BIOSIMILARS & BIOLOGICS

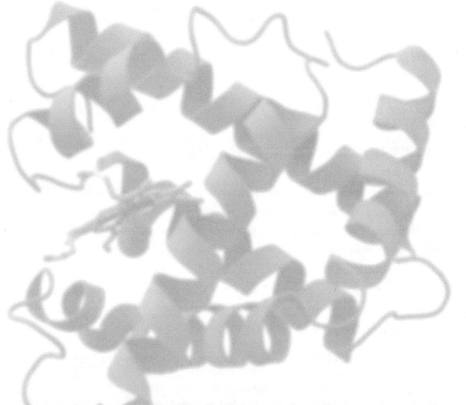

STEVEN LUCIO, PharmD, BCPS

Associate Vice President
Vizient
Irving, Texas

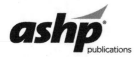

Any correspondence regarding this publication should be sent to the publisher, American Society of Health-System Pharmacists, 4500 East-West Highway, Suite 900, Bethesda, MD 20814, attention: Special Publishing.

The information presented herein reflects the opinions of the contributors and advisors. It should not be interpreted as an official policy of ASHP or as an endorsement of any product.

Because of ongoing research and improvements in technology, the information and its applications contained in this text are constantly evolving and are subject to the professional judgment and interpretation of the practitioner due to the uniqueness of a clinical situation. The editors and ASHP have made reasonable efforts to ensure the accuracy and appropriateness of the information presented in this document. However, any user of this information is advised that the editors and ASHP are not responsible for the continued currency of the information, for any errors or omissions, and/or for any consequences arising from the use of the information in the document in any and all practice settings. Any reader of this document is cautioned that ASHP makes no representation, guarantee, or warranty, express or implied, as to the accuracy and appropriateness of the information contained in this document and specifically disclaims any liability to any party for the accuracy and/or completeness of the material or for any damages arising out of the use or non-use of any of the information contained in this document.

Acquisitions Editor: Beth Campbell

Editorial Project Manager, Special Publishing: Ruth Bloom

Editorial Project Manager, Production: Bill Fogle

Cover & Page Design: David Wade

Page Production: Carol Barrer

Library of Congress Cataloging - in - Publication Data

Names: Lucio, Steven, author.

Title: Biosimilars and biologics : implementation and monitoring in a healthcare setting / Steven Lucio.

Description: Bethesda, MD : American Society of Health-System Pharmacists, Inc., [2018] | Includes bibliographical references and index.

Identifiers: LCCN 2017058790 | ISBN 9781585285808 (pbk.)

Subjects: | MESH: Biosimilar Pharmaceuticals | Drug Compounding | Drug Monitoring

Classification: LCC RM301.25 | NLM QV 241 | DDC 615.1/9--dc23 LC record available at https://lccn.loc.gov/2017058790

© 2018, American Society of Health-System Pharmacists, Inc. All rights reserved.

No part of this publication may be reproduced or transmitted in any form or by any means, electronic or mechanical, including photocopying, microfilming, and recording, or by any information storage and retrieval system, without written permission from the American Society of Health-System Pharmacists.

ASHP is a service mark of the American Society of Health-System Pharmacists, Inc.; registered in the U.S. Patent and Trademark Office.

ISBN: 978-1-58528-580-8

10 9 8 7 6 5 4 3 2 1

DEDICATION

This book is dedicated to

my wife, Jennifer,

for her love, support, and excellent editing skills.

TABLE OF CONTENTS

Preface vii

CHAPTER 1: A New Type of Blockbuster: The Growth of Biologics 1

CHAPTER 2: Déjà vu or Something New?—Comparing the Generic and
Biosimilar Experiences 11

CHAPTER 3: Bugs and Drugs, and Yeast and Mice, and Chinese Hamsters 21

CHAPTER 4: The $250 Billion Pyramid: Analytics in Biosimilarity Determination 33

CHAPTER 5: The Global Biosimilars Experience 57

CHAPTER 6: The American Biosimilar Experience: Red, White, and
Possibly Interchangeable 71

CHAPTER 7: Biosimilar Clinical Trial Requirements 91

CHAPTER 8: Immunogenicity and Pharmacovigilance in the Biosimilar Era 113

CHAPTER 9: The Patent Dance and the Exclusivity Shuffle 127

CHAPTER 10: Defining Biosimilar Value and Other Seemingly Impossible Tasks 139

CHAPTER 11: Biosimilar Formulary Management Strategies 153

CONCLUSION: Biosimilars 2023 167

Index 171

PREFACE

To those reading this text, I thank you for your purchase and for entrusting your time and attention to this book. Hopefully, you find this reference thorough and accessible as you work to define the role of biosimilars within your organizations.

Over the course of reviewing and evaluating the biosimilar concept, three words are likely to come to mind: *complexity, uncertainty,* and *expectation*.

- First, biologic medications, biosimilars and originators alike, are complex molecules in terms of their physicochemical attributes, manufacturing, licensing, regulation, and marketing. As a result, we must fully understand the impact of each of these elements on the implementation of biosimilars into practice.

- Second, many aspects of the regulation, marketing, and financing of the biosimilar model remain uncertain and will continue to evolve. In both of these ways, biosimilars very much resemble the environment into which they are being born as the U.S. health-care system is exceedingly complex, and many aspects about its functioning, including its sustainability, remain uncertain or in some cases are increasing in uncertainty.

- Third, it is an absolutely appropriate expectation for the U.S. biosimilars' process to result in highly similar biologic drugs of comparable safety and efficacy to the originator reference products against which they are compared. Similarly, it is also a reasonable expectation that the introduction of competition will exert downward pressure on the cost of branded biologics and help avert indefinite price escalation of commonly prescribed medications. However, biosimilars should not be expected to correct all of the existing problems that currently confront the healthcare environment or immediately reverse the escalation of drug prices. We must not hold out unrealistic ideals for biosimilar value and in doing so miss the realizable contributions these agents can offer.

Adoption of biosimilars to the extent required to influence market conditions will require a robust and sustained commitment on the part of all stakeholders. Market, legal, regulatory, and practice hurdles exist and will take time to overcome. As such, the work of expanding our understanding of biosimilar development and regulation cannot wait until the market is fully formed but must grow with each incremental step that takes place. This reference is intended to illuminate expected challenges and provide the background pharmacists need to develop strategies to address and minimize these obstacles.

Finally, while biosimilars will not rectify every problem of pharmaceutical supply and expense, we should view the exercise of their introduction in terms broader than simply the addition of competition to the biologics environment. As will be shown throughout this text, appreciating the biosimilar paradigm involves not only a recognition of the elements unique to these biologics, but also an improved awareness of the factors that drive the manufacture, regulation, marketing, distribution, and financing of all pharmaceuticals. For example, quality manufacturing is essential to the accurate structure and functioning of all biologics and is the subject of exceptional scrutiny in the licensing of biosimilars. Given that we continue to face a crisis of drug shortages for generic medications—many due to manufacturing problems—the biosimilar experience should increase our awareness of how essential quality production is to a stable supply of pharmaceuticals.

As a result, I hope this text increases your perspective on biosimilars and other critical elements of pharmaceutical supply.

Best wishes as you embark on your individual journeys in bringing greater rationalization of cost into your practice settings.

Steven Lucio

2018

BIOSIMILARS
& BIOLOGICS

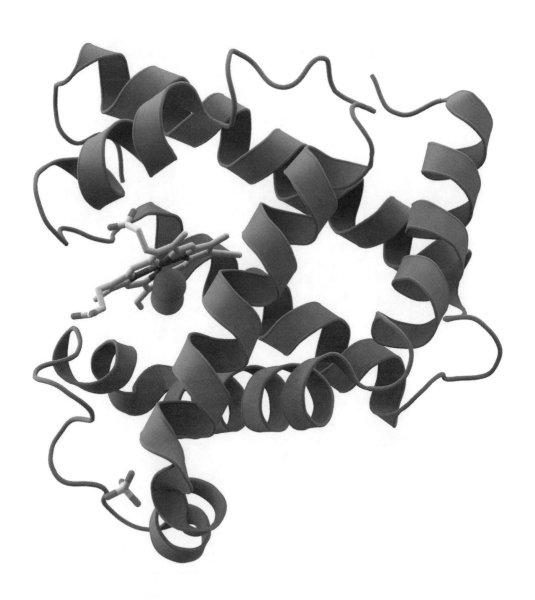

CHAPTER 1

A NEW TYPE OF BLOCKBUSTER: THE GROWTH OF BIOLOGICS

A recent industry report noted that approximately 35 proposed biosimilar versions of eight of the most commonly prescribed U.S. biologic drugs have achieved Phase III clinical trial status or proceeded even further toward final approval.[1] In addition, another 27 biosimilar candidates of these same molecules remain in pre-clinical or Phase I testing.[1] Although the estimated development costs for each biosimilar range from $100 million to $250 million,[2] this financial commitment has not deterred a substantial number of aspiring manufacturers that view the ability to replicate and market highly similar versions of originator biologics as a desirable and ideally lucrative competency. This degree of investment is a direct result of the extraordinary influence biologic drugs have exerted on the pharmaceutical and healthcare landscape over the previous three decades.[3] The availability of biologic medications has transformed the management of many critical diseases, offered significantly improved outcomes for patients, and redefined expectations for drug development success and return on investment.[3-5] Like their small molecule predecessors, the success and acceptance of branded biologics has created not just the opportunity, but also the critical need for competition and associated financial savings.[2] To appreciate the unique characteristics that will define the biosimilars market, we must first understand how biologic drugs have altered the treatment landscape.

FROM INSULIN TO IMMUNOTHERAPY

Few could have predicted that the recombinant technology revolution would affect such financial success for the pharmaceutical industry and the extent of patient benefit. However, that is exactly what has transpired following the Food and Drug Administration's (FDA) approval of the first recombinant biologic product, human insulin (Humulin) in 1982 (**Table 1-1**).[3] Created by Genentech and marketed by Eli Lilly, the introduction of recombinant human insulin revolutionized the treatment of diabetes by making a replica of this human protein to minimize the likelihood of adverse events associated with bovine- or porcine-derived products and to ensure a more stable and sustainable manufacturing process.[3] Since then, recombinant technology has been utilized to produce not only copies of existing, naturally occurring insulin, but also specifically engineered versions that enable either a more rapid onset of action or a prolonged coverage to meet basal requirements.[4] Recombinant biologics now define a fundamental component of care not only for diabetes, but also for oncology conditions, rheumatoid arthritis, inflammatory bowel diseases, immunology, and cardiovascular illnesses.[4,5]

TABLE 1-1. Key Milestones in Recombinant Biologic Development[3,5-8]

Date	Product	Indication	Importance
1982	Recombinant human insulin	Diabetes	First recombinant biologic approved
1986	Muromonab-CD3[a]	Prevention of organ rejection	First approved monoclonal antibody; murine antibody
1989	Epoetin	Treatment of anemia	First erythropoietin approved
1991	Filgrastim	Chemotherapy induced neutropenia	First colony stimulating factor approved
1993	Abciximab	Glycoprotein IIb/IIIa antiplatelet therapy	First approved, chimeric monoclonal antibody
1997	Daclizumab[a]	Anti-rejection drug	First approved, humanized monoclonal antibody
1998	Infliximab	Biologic disease modifying anti-rheumatic drug	First approved, tumor necrosis factor inhibitor (chimeric antibody)
2002	Adalimumab	Biologic disease modifying anti-rheumatic drug	First approved, fully human monoclonal antibody
2011	Ipilimumab	Treatment of melanoma	First approved, monoclonal antibody immunotherapy
2014	Pembrolizumab	Treatment of melanoma, skin cancer	First approved, monoclonal antibody program cell death-1 (PD-1) inhibitor
2015	Alirocumab	Treatment of hypercholesterolemia	First approved, monoclonal antibody against proprotein convertase subtilisin kexin type 9 (PCSK9)
2016	Atezolizumab	Bladder cancer	First approved, monoclonal antibody programmed death ligand 1 (PD-L1) inhibitor

[a]Product no longer marketed in the United States.

Biologics remain a critical component of new drug development as evidenced by their expansion into novel areas of treatment such as immunotherapy agents, like the program cell death (PD-1) and programmed death ligand 1 (PD-L1) inhibitors.[6,8] Similarly, biologics provide new approaches to established treatment areas with products such as the proprotein convertase subtilisin kexin type 9 (PCSK9) inhibitors in hypercholesterolemia.[6-8] This degree of innovation is seen not only in these specific products, but also for biologics as a whole. In an analysis of new molecular entities approved between 1986 and 2014, biologic drugs were more likely to be first-in-class products (54% versus 24%) as compared to their small molecule counterparts and less likely (26% versus 49%) to be addition-to-class medications with no clinical advantage over existing therapies.[9]

Given this success and extent of therapeutic advancement, it is no surprise that many biologic drugs have achieved the designation of blockbuster medications, generally defined as products with greater than $1 billion in sales.[10] Although many small molecule medications have also achieved this threshold, the influence of biologics is particularly evident when evaluating the top spend medications across the United States.[1]

THE BIOLOGIC BLOCKBUSTER

The influence of biologics as top spend drugs has continued to expand in recent years. As seen in **Table 1-2**, only one biologic product, epoetin alfa, registered among the top 10 medications in use in 2010.[11] In 2016, five of the top 10 medications were biologic drugs.[12] Also, in 2010, that lone biologic, epoetin, accounted for $3.3 billion.[11] In 2016, the five biologic agents among the top 10 represented over $36 billion.[12]

As small molecule blockbusters like atorvastatin, esomeprazole, clopidogrel, quetiapine, montelukast, and most recently, rosuvastatin have reached the end of their exclusivities, numerous biologic products now occupy their positions as top spend drugs.[1,12] However, the type of product (i.e., biologic versus small molecule) is only one difference in the profiles of these medications. There are also variations between current and previous blockbusters in terms of the

TABLE 1-2. Top U.S. Prescription Drugs (2010 versus 2016)[11-13]

2010			2016		
Total Spend = $307.4 billion			Total Spend = $450 billion		
Rank	Drug Name	Total Sales (billions)	Rank	Drug Name	Total Sales (billions)
1	Atorvastatin (Lipitor)	$7.2	**1**	**Adalimumab (Humira)**	$13.6
2	Esomeprazole (Nexium)	$6.3	2	Ledipasvir/sofosbuvir (Harvoni)	$10.0
3	Clopidogrel (Plavix)	$6.1	3	**Etanercept (Enbrel)**	$7.4
4	Salmeterol/Fluticasone (Advair Diskus)	$4.7	**4**	**Insulin glargine[a] (Lantus Solostar)**	$5.7
5	Aripiprazole (Abilify)	$4.6	5	**Infliximab (Remicade)**	$5.3
6	Quetiapine (Seroquel)	$4.4	6	Sitagliptin	$4.8
7	Montelukast (Singulair)	$4.1	7	Salmeterol/Fluticasone (Advair Diskus)	$4.7
8	Rosuvastatin (Crestor)	$3.8	8	Pregabalin (Lyrica)	$4.4
9	Pioglitazone (Actos)	$3.5	9	Rosuvastatin (Crestor)	$4.2
10	**Epoetin alfa (Epogen)**	$3.3	**10**	**Pegfilgrastim (Neulasta)**	$4.2
Other Top Recombinant Biologic Drugs in the Top 20					
11	**Infliximab (Remicade)**	$3.3	12	**Rituximab (Rituxan)**	$3.9
12	**Etanercept (Enbrel)**	$3.3	15	**Insulin glargine[a] (Lantus)**	$3.3
14	**Bevacizumab (Avastin)**	$3.1	19	**Bevacizumab (Avastin)**	$3.1
16	**Pegfilgrastim (Neulasta)**	$3.0			
18	**Adalimumab (Humira)**	$2.9			
20	**Rituximab (Rituxan)**	$2.8			

Drugs in boldface = recombinant biologic products.

[a]Currently regulated as a small molecule drug; however, will be considered a biologic after March 23, 2020.

size of the patient population served by these agents, their individual costs, and the rigor applied to their management.

A NEW BLOCKBUSTER EQUATION (COST IS INVERSELY PROPORTIONAL TO THE POPULATION TREATED)

The Narrowing of Patient Populations

Historically, the products most likely to achieve blockbuster status and drive the greatest degree of sales were those agents used across the largest patient populations.[10] The more patients served, the more prescriptions written, and the greater the volume of medications dispensed. Innovation within the small molecule world has provided numerous, now generically sourced, treatment alternatives for common conditions such as hypertension, high cholesterol, depression, gastrointestinal disorders, cardiovascular diseases, and allergies, just to list a few.[10] Given this extent of success, in terms of clinical advancement followed by robust generic competition, fewer primary care–focused medications now drive blockbuster sales. In 2000, approximately 90% of blockbusters were directed toward primary care conditions.[10] By 2010, this percentage had decreased closer to 60%.[10] Conversely, the percentage of blockbusters that were biologics increased from approximately 10% to 30% over that same period.[10] In 2010, top selling drugs such as clopidogrel, atorvastatin, and montelukast were used in patient populations of 5.1 million, 4.8 million, and 3.6 million, respectively.[14] In contrast, in 2014, top selling biologic drugs adalimumab, etanercept, and infliximab were used in approximately 245,000, 224,000, and 278,000 patients, respectively.[14] A recent estimate suggests that 42% of products in the investigational pipeline, both small molecule and biologic, will be specialty medications.[15] Therefore, in contrast to the previous era, blockbuster medications now are frequently identified by their degree of specialization for a very targeted patient population including ultra-specialized drugs (i.e., orphan drugs).[14,16] This narrowing of the patient audience for new drugs, both small molecules and biologics, correlates with another critical issue, medication costs.

The Relative Cost of Biologics

The most recent estimated cost for developing a novel medication is $2.6 billion.[17] If a new medication is intended for a very common condition, there are many patients and associated dispensed prescriptions over which the development costs could be distributed. However, as many new products are increasingly intended for specialized conditions, the number of patients who could benefit from the drug and drive revenue is smaller.[14] In addition, biologic drugs are associated with more expense due to the cost of acquiring the expertise and establishing the technology to support recombinant manufacturing.[14] Unlike small molecule medications, which can in some cases be administered orally, biologic drugs are limited to parenteral delivery, which can necessitate special handling and administration requirements.[18] These dosage forms, coupled with more rigorous storage conditions and the skill set to administer and monitor them, also contribute to their expense.[18] Prior to the 2012 patent cliff, the two top selling medications were clopidogrel and atorvastatin.[11,14] Both of these products had reached a point in their lifecycle where their annual costs were $1,900 (or $160 monthly).[19] In contrast, a 2012 analysis of managed care data revealed an annual treatment cost of tumor necrosis factor–alpha inhibitors, frequently prescribed biologics, of $15,345, $18,046; and $24,018 for etanercept, adalimumab, and infliximab, respectively.[20]

Many market factors beyond the cost of drug development and administration contribute to the ultimate price of a medication.[14] The new hepatitis C therapies have reinforced the fact that high treatment costs are not limited to biologic medications.[1,12] However, biologic therapies in general have a higher relative cost and, more importantly, were previously protected from price lowering competition.[15]

BIOLOGIC IMMUNITY—FROM COMPETITION

Indefinite Exclusivity

A critical aspect of the pharmacy supply chain is the fact that innovation is rewarded through a period of patent protection and exclusivity.[21] However, once that timeframe has expired, other manufacturers can synthesize the same molecule, thus allowing for competition and ideally increasing access to a therapeutic standard of care. Prior to the introduction of biosimilars, this process did not exist for the vast majority of the biologic pharmaceutical environment.[13] As a result, commonly used biologics have not only achieved blockbuster status, but have also endured as top spend medications for extended, and until recently, indefinite periods of time.[1,11,12]

Figures 1-1 and **1-2** illustrate the differences between small molecule medications and biologics in terms of the duration of exclusivity. As can been seen in **Figure 1-3**, the period of exclusivity for blockbuster small molecules has been 12 to 15 years.[11,22] A recent analysis of top selling prescription drugs that experienced generic competition between 2000 and 2012 revealed a median effective market exclusivity period of 12.5 years.[23] Drugs that were either first in their class or represented an advancement had longer exclusivity periods of 14.5 years and 14.3 years, respectively.[23]

Upon its approval in 2010, the Biologics Price Competition and Innovation (BPCI) Act set the duration of exclusivity for originator reference biologics at 12 years.[13] During this window, the FDA cannot approve a competing biosimilar.[13] As will be described in Chapter 9, patent issues

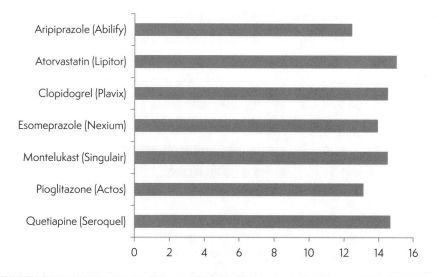

FIGURE 1-1. RELATIVE YEARS OF EXCLUSIVITY FOR RECENT SMALL MOLECULE BLOCK-BUSTER DRUGS.[11,22]

also impact the timing of competition launch.[24] Therefore, biosimilar competition will not necessarily arrive exactly 12 years after the date of initial approval of the originator branded biologic. As can be seen below (Figure 1-2), many commonly prescribed biologics were approved long before the BPCI Act went into effect and have existed without competition well over 12 years.

The top selling biologics—filgrastim, infliximab, etanercept, adalimumab, and bevacizumab—now have FDA-approved biosimilar competitors.[22] However, patent litigation issues continue to delay the launch of several of these approved products further lengthening the effective exclusivity of their originator counterparts.[25] Another biologic, epoetin, has achieved almost 30 years of exclusivity without competition from a different manufacturer, although that window finally appears to be closing as an anticipated biosimilar is continuing to work its way through the regulatory process.[26]

Given the lower development costs of generics, it is not uncommon for multiple suppliers to enter the market upon loss of exclusivity or shortly thereafter.[2,22] The biosimilar paradigm is much different. Given the more rigorous analytical and clinical filing requirements and financial commitments, biosimilars even of the same molecule will not necessarily enter the application and submission phase at the same time.[2,13,22] Due to these differences in approval and litigation time requirements, multiple biosimilars for the same reference biologic will enter the market in a staggered fashion, creating a more stepwise accrual of pricing discounts and savings opportunities.[27]

The Financial Consequences of Prolonged Exclusivity

Price increases of pharmaceuticals are usually arrested and reversed with the introduction of generic competition. The absence of this process for biologics was recently articulated in an analysis of the annualized percentage price increase for top biologic drugs purchased in the United States.[28] In some circumstances, particularly for versions of interferon beta-1a (Avonex;

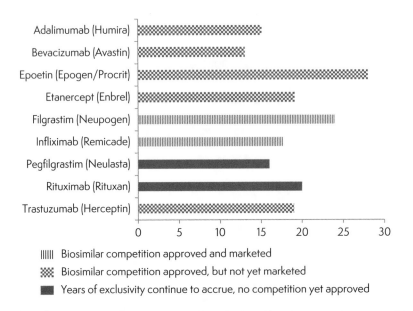

FIGURE 1-2. RELATIVE YEARS OF EXCLUSIVITY FOR COMMON ORIGINATOR REFERENCE BIOLOGICS.[11,22]

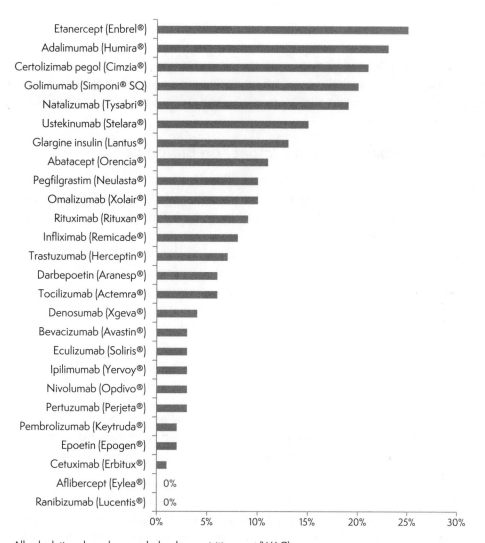

All calculations based upon wholesale acquisition cost (WAC).

FIGURE 1-3. ANNUAL AVERAGE PRICE INCREASES FOR TOP BIOLOGIC PURCHASED DRUGS.[28,29]

Biogen and Rebif; EMD Serono) used in the treatment of multiple sclerosis, the annualized average percentage price increase was 36% and 35%, respectively.[28] For the top biologics where biosimilar competition already exists or is nearing final approval and marketing, annualized price increases from initial launch until present were: infliximab, 8%; etanercept, 25%; adalimumab, 23%, pegfilgrastim, 10%; and trastuzumab, 7%.[28] Figure 1-3 shows the percentage increases for commonly prescribed biologics.[28,29]

Obviously, not all biologic products have exhibited the same degree of increase. For example, two medications for macular degeneration, aflibercept and ranibizumab, have maintained a rather static price.[28,29] It should be noted that these two products are competitors along with another top biologic, bevacizumab, which is used off-label in this indication.[30] The presence of effective, therapeutic alternatives may have helped moderate more aggressive price increases for this biologic category. Also, providers usually participate in programs that offer discounts and/or rebates and ultimately pay something less than the wholesale acquisition cost (WAC) or list price.[1,12] Still, such discounts are usually in the range of a few percentage points and do not completely erase routine price increases.[1,12] As a result, direct competition following loss of exclusivity is necessary.

The Specialty Pharmacy Era's Impact on Biologics

One of the most critical distinctions between the blockbuster experience for generic drugs as compared to biosimilars is how these products are managed, delivered, dispensed, and monitored. For most small molecule blockbusters, the introduction of generic versions allows rapid uptake regardless of the site of care, given the familiarity with the products, the ease of substitution, and the lack of an extensive formulary analysis.[2] Due to the issues described above, particularly the relative costs of therapy and the narrow patient populations treated, biologic drug prescribing has invited a greater degree of scrutiny by managed care organizations, who control the payment for therapy, and healthcare providers, who must frequently administer and monitor biologic treatment.[31] With the exception of the insulin products, payers, including the pharmacy benefit management companies responsible for managing drug expenditures, view biologic drugs as specialty products.[32] These organizations attempt to manage drug utilization and cost through strategies such as prior authorization requirements, step therapy, partial fills, higher co-pays/co-insurance, and limited access through predefined specialty pharmacy channels.[31] In addition to the cost and special handling requirements of parenteral agents, some of which cannot be self-administered, the intervention of providers, physicians, and healthcare institutions is required to ensure safe and appropriate preparation and delivery, coupled with close monitoring.[18]

Rather than a circumstance where use of generics is primarily determined at the level of prescribing or dispensing, the choice of biosimilars will be directed, incentivized, and rigorously monitored at a higher organizational level. Managed care entities have already initiated the preferential placement of biosimilars on their formularies.[33] Similarly, numerous health-system pharmacy and therapeutics committees have started to assess and identify preferred agents.[34] The good news is that biosimilars can be integrated into the formulary management infrastructures that already exist for their branded biologic counterparts.[34] However, this work of integration will require substantial resource and time commitment. Biosimilars will challenge manufacturers to meet these organizations' expectations in terms of the clinical understanding and meaningful value propositions needed to prompt a conversion from an originator biologic.[2]

KEY POINTS

- Recombinant biologic products have revolutionized the treatment of many diseases and drive a substantial amount of expense for the healthcare landscape.

- The initial higher cost of biologic drugs, their specialized patient populations, and the absence of competition have all contributed to greater expense for these product categories.

- Biosimilar competition is critical to managing pharmaceutical expense given the impact of biologics on current and anticipated costs.

CONCLUSION

Biologic drugs have more than earned their designation as blockbuster medications due to the many treatments that have redefined the standard of care and improved the quality of life for countless patients. However, this degree of success has come at a substantial price (literally) given the expense that accompanies these agents, heightening the need for competition. In the absence of biosimilars, the cost of biologic medications would continue to escalate, creating additional barriers to access not only for existing therapies, but also for the novel and improved treatments under development. The success and costs of biologic blockbusters have also contributed to an entirely new supply chain for expensive agents—the specialty pharmacy channel. To achieve meaningful use, biosimilars must be integrated into this infrastructure as viable alternatives to long-established brands.

REFERENCES

1. IMS Health. Medicines use and spending in the U.S.—a review of 2015 and outlook to 2020, April 2016. www.imshealth.com/en/thought-leadership/quintilesims-institute/reports/medicines-use-and-spending-in-the-us-a-review-of-2015-and-outlook-to-2020 (accessed 3 Oct 2017).
2. Blackstone EA, Fuhr JP. The economics of biosimilars. *Am Health Drug Benefits.* 2013; 6:469-78.
3. Kinch MS. An overview of FDA-approved biologics medicines. *Drug Discov Today.* 2015; 20:393-8.
4. Tibaldi JM. Evolution of insulin: from human to analog. *Am J Med.* 2014; 127(10 Suppl):S25-38.
5. Ecker DM, Jones SD, Levine HL. The therapeutic monoclonal antibody market. *MAbs* 2015; 7:9-14.
6. Keytruda (pembrolizumab) package insert. Whitehouse Station, NJ: Merck & Co., Inc.; 2016.
7. Praluent (alirocumab) package insert. Bridewater, NJ: Sanofi-Aventis U.S.; 2015.
8. Tecentriq (atezolizumab) package insert. South San Francisco, CA: Genentech, Inc; 2016.
9. Miller KL, Lanthier M. Regulatory watch: innovation in biologic new molecular entities: 1986-2014. *Nat Rev Drug Discov.* 2015; 14:83.
10. Jacquet P, Schwarzbach E, Oren I. The new face of blockbuster drugs. IN VIVO. 2011; 29:2-7.
11. IMS Health. The use of medicines in the United States: Review of 2010, April 2011. www.imshealth.com/files/web/IMSH%20Institute/Reports/The%20Use%20of%20Medicines%20in%20the%20United%20States%202010/Use_of_Meds_in_the_U.S._Review_of_2010.pdf (accessed 3 Oct 2017).
12. QuintilesIMS. Medicines use and spending in the U.S. A review of 2016 and Outlook to 2021. www.imshealth.com/en/thought-leadership/quintilesims-institute/reports/medicines-use-and-spending-in-the-us-review-of-2016-outlook-to-2021 (accessed 3 Oct 2017).
13. Title VII: Improving access to innovative medical therapies. Subtitle A: Biologic Price Competition and Innovation provisions of the Patient Protection and Affordable Care Act (PPACA). www.fda.gov/downloads/Drugs/GuidanceComplianceRegulatoryInformation/ucm216146.pdf (accessed 3 Oct 2017).
14. EvaluatePharma. Budget-Busters: The shift to high-priced innovator drugs in the USA. September 2014. www.info.evaluategroup.com/rs/evaluatepharmaltd/images/SV2014.pdf (accessed 3 Oct 2017).
15. Purvis L, Kuntz C. Is high prescription drug spending becoming our new normal? Health Affairs Blog. www.healthaffairs.org/blog/2016/05/17/is-high-prescription-drug-spending-becoming-our-new-normal/ (accessed 3 Oct 2017).
16. Liao J, Pauly M. Orphan drugs: pursuing value and avoiding unintended effects of regulations. Health Affairs Blog. www.healthaffairs.org/blog/2017/05/04/orphan-drugs-pursuing-value-and-avoiding-unintended-effects-of-regulations/ (accessed 3 Oct 2017).

17. DiMasi JA, Grabowski HG, Hansen RW. Innovation in the pharmaceutical industry: new estimates of R & D costs. *J Health Econ.* 2016; 47:20-33.

18. Morrow T, Felcone LH. Defining the difference: what makes biologics unique. *Biotechnol Healthc.* 2004; 1:24-6.

19. DeRuiter J, Holston PL. Drug patent expirations and the "patent cliff." *U.S. Pharm.* 2012; 37(generic suppl):12-20. www.uspharmacist.com/article/drug-patent-expirations-and-the-patent-cliff (accessed 3 Oct 2017).

20. Bonafede MM, Gandra SR, Watson C et al. Cost per treated patient for etanercept, adaliumumab, and infliximab across adult indications: a claims analysis. *Adv Ther.* 2012; 29:234-48.

21. Kesselheim AS, Avorn J, Sarpatwari A. The high cost of prescription drugs in the United States: Origins and prospects for reform. *JAMA.* 2016; 316:858-71.

22. Drugs@FDA: FDA approved drug products database. www.fda.gov/Drugs/InformationOnDrugs/ucm135821.htm (accessed Feb. 26, 2018).

23. Wang B, Liu J, Kesselheim AS. Variations in time of market exclusivity among top-selling prescription drugs in the United States. *JAMA Intern Med.* 2015; 175:635-7.

24. Mehr SR. Pharmaceutical patent litigation and the emerging biosimilars: a conversation with Kevin M. Nelson, JD. *Am Health Drug Benefits.* 2017; 10:23-6.

25. Barlas S. Early biosimilars face hurdles to acceptance: the FDA has approved few, so lack of competition is keeping prices high. *P T.* 2016; 41:362-5.

26. Palmer E. FDA rejects Pfizer's Epogen biosimilar for the second time. www.fiercepharma.com/regulatory/fda-rejects-pfizer-s-epogen-biosimilar-for-a-second-time (accessed 3 Oct 2017).

27. Big Molecule Watch. BPCIA litigation summary chart. www.bigmoleculewatch.com/bpcia-litigation-summary-chart/ (accessed 3 Oct 2017).

28. Huggett B. America's drug problem. *Nat Biotechnol.* 2016; 34:1231-41.

29. Medi-Span Price Rx Pro database (subscription) (accessed 23 July 2017).

30. Age-related Macular Degeneration Preferred Practice Patterns. American Academy of Ophthalmology. www.aao.org/preferred-practice-pattern/age-related-macular-degeneration-ppp-2015 (accessed 3 Oct 2017).

31. EMD Serono Specialty Digest, 13th edition, 2017. www.specialtydigestemdserono.com/ (accessed 3 Oct 2017).

32. Express Scripts 2016 Drug Trend Report, February 2017. www.lab.express-scripts.com/lab/drug-trend-report (accessed 3 Oct 2017).

33. CVS Health. 2017 Standard Formulary List of Removals and Updates. www.investors.cvshealth.com/~/media/Files/C/CVS-IR-v3/documents/02-aug-2016/2017-standard-formulary-list-of-removals-and-updates.pdf (accessed 3 Oct 2017).

34. Traynor K. Filgrastim becomes biosimilar test case for hospitals. *Am J Health Syst Pharm.* 2016; 73:1805-6.

CHAPTER 2

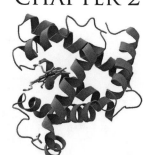

DÉJÀ VU OR SOMETHING NEW?—COMPARING THE GENERIC AND BIOSIMILAR EXPERIENCES

Drug products from different sources may differ in quality in several respects. These differences, individually, or collectively, may lead to substantial differences in therapeutic effect and/or safety.

> Not only may the products of different manufacturers vary, but the product of a single manufacturer may vary from batch to batch...

> With the emphasis currently being placed upon cost containment in all areas of healthcare and the increasing numbers of important drugs for which patents are expiring, it seems clear that pressure to substitute a cheaper product for the one prescribed will increase.[1]

The above comments appear to reflect common perceptions and apprehensions regarding the use of biosimilars and their role in therapy. First, some healthcare providers remain unsure about how to interpret the inherent variability of biologics and the potential impact of this characteristic on the clinical safety and efficacy of biosimilars. Clinicians continue to express concern about the degree to which regulatory statutes, practice guidelines, and formulary determinations will preferentially recommend the use of biosimilars and/or encourage their substitution in place of originator reference products. Finally, the principal justification for biosimilar development and adoption is an economic one, prompting concern of how the opportunity for savings will be balanced with the goal of delivering high quality medication therapy.

Interestingly, the above comments are in fact not about biosimilars, but instead demonstrate the apprehension of physicians, pharmacists, and other clinicians toward the safety and efficacy of generic medications.[1] These statements from the *American Journal of Medicine* (August 23, 1985) reveal that the generic paradigm did not find immediate acceptance and integration into medical practice, but instead faced many similar challenges to those that currently confront the emerging biosimilars market.[1] With up to 89% of prescriptions now filled with generic medications (**Table 2-1**), we can conclude that much of this initial apprehension has been overcome in the intervening 30+ years since the implementation of the Drug Price Competition and Patent Term Restoration Act of 1984 (i.e., Hatch-Waxman), which defined the modern approach to competition for small molecule medications.[2]

TABLE 2-1. Percentage of Prescriptions Filled with Generic Drugs[2,3]

Year	Percentage
1984	19%
1990	33%
1996	43%
2002	53%
2008	72%
2013	86%
2015	89%

As we look toward the biosimilars market following the enactment of the Biologics Price Competition and Innovation Act (i.e., the biosimilars act), the question persists as to the extent we can replicate the success of generics and how much of an educational and advocacy investment will be required to attain a similarly high degree of acceptance. In addition, what can we learn from the generic experience to assist us in building a robust market for highly similar biologics to drive down costs to providers, payers, and most of all patients? As we will see, some aspects of the infrastructure that facilitated generic adoption will also enable the use of biosimilars. However, other challenges will be completely unique, due not only to the characteristics of biologics, but also the way in which the healthcare landscape has evolved.

THE GENERIC EXPERIENCE

For those new to healthcare practice, it seems unthinkable that the concept of generic medications was ever considered novel, much less viewed with a high degree of suspicion and concern. Nevertheless, that situation is exactly the dynamic into which the generic era was born. In the initial years subsequent to Hatch-Waxman, physicians and pharmacists questioned foundational elements of the Abbreviated New Drug Application (ANDA) pathway including the definition of bioequivalence, the therapeutic equivalency rating of generic products with their branded reference counterparts, and the general aspects of the approval process (**Table 2-2**).[1,4,5]

Addressing this uncertainty required significant time and investment for the Food and Drug Administration (FDA) not only to develop the infrastructure to support ANDA review, but also to explain and defend the methodology of generic approval to physicians and pharmacists.[6-8] The efforts of branded manufacturers to build on prescribers' concerns through aggressive anti-generic marketing efforts far beyond the product detailing we see today made this task more difficult.[6] In addition, FDA even endured a scandal involving certain generic manufacturers filing fraudulent applications and bribing officials within the Division of Generic Drugs to expedite the review of ANDAs.[6,8] These activities increased the level of suspicion of generic medications and slowed adoption for several years.[6,8] It is encouraging to note that despite these challenges the generic concept succeeded through the FDA's efforts to increase public confidence and to build in safeguards to protect the integrity of the review process.[6,8] Still, the greatest force for adoption was the need for cost savings. The rising cost of healthcare, the increase in the demand

TABLE 2-2. Initial Issues and Concerns with Generic Drugs[4,5]

Issues	Concerns
Provider and patient choice	■ Substitution without providers' or patients' knowledge ■ Mandated substitution or switching ■ Restriction of product availability
Legal issues	■ FDA perceived favoritism towards generics ■ Legal challenges ■ Liability issues
FDA methodology	■ Unilaterally created internal guidance and its flexibility versus regulations ■ Absence of requirement for new clinical data ■ Confidence in abbreviated approach to determination of equivalence
Market factors	■ Initial savings less than predicted ■ Generic medication not always less expensive than the brand

FDA = Food and Drug Administration.

for prescription drugs, and the emergence of managed care organizations collectively helped erode much of the fear and uncertainty about generic medications.[6]

During the generics era, the role of managed care organizations and their influence on mitigating prescription drug expenses became more prominent. Through formulary management strategies and incentives such as tiering and co-payment programs, managed care organizations encouraged the use of preferred types of drug products, such as generic medications.[6] A similar level of success was realized in the inpatient arena, where hospitals focused prescribing to include a maximization of generic use wherever possible.[6] In both settings, the substitutability made possible through FDA's therapeutic equivalence or "Orange Book" rating greatly enhanced the ease of adoption.[8] Economic necessity coupled with the ease of substitution simplified the pathway for generic acceptance.[6,8]

WHAT FROM THE GENERIC EXPERIENCE APPLIES TO BIOSIMILARS?

The High Cost of Drugs

Although not good news for the healthcare environment in general, the seemingly exponential growth in drug prices continues to drive a search for any and all cost savings opportunities, which ideally should create a fertile environment for biosimilars. In 1980, four years prior to the advent of Hatch-Waxman, $11 billion was spent on prescription drugs in the United States.[9] In 2016, the annual spend on prescription medications was $450 billion, and current projections suggest that figure could exceed $600 billion by 2021, an amount comparable to the size of the U.S. defense budget.[10,11] The continual criticism of higher prices for all drugs, new and old, small molecule and biologic, illustrates the providers', payers', the government's, and the public's desperation to seek some measure of relief.[11]

The availability and use of generics resulted in an estimated $1.5 trillion in savings from 2005 to 2015 (**Table 2-3**).[2] Fewer blockbuster generic opportunities are anticipated in the near term, given the influence of biologic drugs as medications with the highest dollar spend. Therefore, the most meaningful loss of exclusivity opportunities will reside within the biosimilar category.[10] Various analyses initially estimated a savings opportunity of anywhere from $13 to $250 billion between 2014 and 2024.[12] However, the continuing legal challenges and delay of product launches following approval could slow the rate of savings realization. Regardless of the actual value, the crisis of pharmaceutical expenditures would appear to provide at least some of the inertia needed to sustain interest and acceptance.

The Growth of Managed Care and Formulary Management Strategies

The biosimilar cause will also benefit from the infrastructure developed to manage the cost of expensive, sole source, branded products.[13-15] As compared to the 1980s, the influence of managed care is more prominent and has now grown to encompass dispensing and delivery of many expensive products (i.e., specialty pharmacy services), especially those targeted for biosimilar development.[13] These organizations will be central to the support of biosimilar adoption and have already taken steps to exclude originator reference biologics from their formularies.[14] Similarly, health-system practices have long honed their skills with the therapeutic interchange of related, yet molecularly distinct medications within targeted drug classes.[15] Even in the absence of an official FDA interchangeability designation, health systems will continue to implement the interchange of biosimilars for originator biologics, as clinically and economically appropriate, based on the oversight of the pharmacy and therapeutics committee of each organization.[15]

TABLE 2-3. Total Annual Savings from Generics (2005 to 2015)[2]

Year	Savings (Billions)
2005	$53
2006	$63
2007	$82
2008	$98
2009	$119
2010	$135
2011	$155
2012	$172
2013	$198
2014	$207
2015	$227

ANOTHER BENEFIT—WE ARE NOT THE FIRST TO THIS PARTY

One additional element that should support the implementation of the biosimilars market in the United States is the fact that other parts of the world, most notably Europe, have already established a lengthy track record with these products.[16] The experience, successes, and failures in the European Union (EU), which will be described in more detail in Chapter 5, can inform our approach here in the United States. In terms of success, over 35 biosimilars have been approved by the European Medicines Agency since 2006, and these agents have demonstrated similar safety and efficacy as compared to their originator counterparts.[16,17] Cost savings and expanded access to care have both been realized.[18] Still, the adoption rate for biosimilars has been slower than desired, and some prescribers continue to view these comparable agents with a degree of concern.[18] In addition, because each country in the EU has taken different approaches to implementation, the adoption rate has varied substantially.[18,19] Countries that define a higher expectation for physician prescribing of biosimilars, and areas where reimbursement aligns with biosimilar use seem to have had greater success with acceptance.[19] All of these examples are extremely insightful for the U.S. experience.

WHAT IS NOT APPLICABLE

Biosimilars Are Not Biogenerics

Although these aspects of the generic market remain relevant for biosimilars, there are also a number of issues that vary substantially, beginning with the unique attributes of biologic drugs. Biologics are inherently more complicated than small molecule medications, are more expensive and more difficult to manufacture, and demonstrate inherent variability (even among the originators).[15] It is for this reason that the pre-existing ANDA pathway was not a viable mechanism for the approval of competing versions of biologics and why it is inaccurate to characterize biosimilars as biogenerics, which would imply an identical copy.[15] As compared to generics, biosimilar licensing is a more involved endeavor that relies on an exhaustive and detailed analytical characterization followed by a clinical data requirement not present in generic approvals.[15]

We Haven't Had 30 Years to Digest These Changes

As a novel approval mechanism, every aspect of the biosimilar pathway is new, even for FDA. Therefore, many of the essential guideposts that have been established through regulation, legal interpretation, or accepted clinical best practice must now be viewed and understood through a different lens. For example, substitutability greatly advanced the ease of generic uptake as most of these medications, upon initial licensing, are designated as therapeutically equivalent or interchangeable with the branded drug.[6,8] In addition, state laws have been modified over time not only to recognize substitution, but also to grant pharmacists the discretion of substituting a generic medication for a branded product without prescriber notification or intervention.[6,20] Although FDA possesses the authority to designate a biosimilar as interchangeable, the requirements to attain this status have only recently been published in draft form.[21] Furthermore, FDA has stated that even with an interchangeability standard established, it is unlikely such a determination could be made upon initial approval for every biosimilar.[21,22] As a result, we would expect biosimilars to be approved and marketed for some period of time without an interchangeability designation. The likelihood of biosimilar manufacturers pursuing this status remains unknown.[15] Currently, numerous states have taken different approaches regarding the recognition of this right to interchange or substitute a biosimilar.[23] The uncertainty around just this one characteristic illustrates the difficulty in fostering a high level of confidence and ease of adoption for biosimilars. This challenge and other critical differences between generics and biosimilars are captured in **Table 2-4**.

Familiarity ≠ Understanding

Although clinicians and patients have come to accept the generic concept, true comprehension of the requirements for approval for these products, much less any prescription medication remains limited.[26,27] Studies have periodically documented the continued latent hesitancy to prescribe generic drugs, particularly in perceived narrow therapeutic index categories, such as anticoagulants, immunosuppressants, and anticonvulsants.[20] A recent study described the lack of familiarity among physicians not only of the approval process for new drugs, but also the specific designations granted to products where preliminary evidence suggests therapeutic benefit over existing treatment options.[25] Therefore, given the confusion and limited appreciation of existing approval standards, introducing another concept, particularly one as nuanced as that of biosimilarity, presents additional challenges.

Savings, But Will It Be Enough?

Finally, the goal of the biosimilar market is to lower the costs of pharmaceuticals. Such value would likely occur, at least in part, through lower prices. Within the generic landscape, pricing concessions of 75% to 90% are not uncommon given the relatively lower expense needed to develop and deliver a generic molecule along with the number of competitors that enter the

TABLE 2-4. Key Operational Differences (Generics Versus Biosimilars)[15,21-25]

Product Characteristic	Generics	Biosimilars
Chemically synthesized and identical to originator	Yes	No
Approval based on bioequivalence alone/no clinical data required	Yes	No
Formulary review not required prior to adoption	Yes	No
Product possesses same generic (i.e., nonproprietary) name as the originator	Yes	No
Product is granted interchangeability (i.e., therapeutic equivalence/ Orange Book rating) with originator at the time of initial approval without additional clinical evidence related to switching between products	Yes	No
Substitution laws in all states define clear and consistent approach to allow for pharmacist interchange of the product for the branded agents prescribed	Yes	No
Prescribers, pharmacists, nurses, patients have reasonable familiarity with concept of competing products	Yes	No
Value proposition clearly defined and understood by all involved stakeholders	Yes	No

market upon branded product loss of exclusivity.[15] As biosimilars require a greater development investment and have a higher cost associated with regulatory approval, discounts are anticipated to be more modest and closer to the 10% to 20% range due to this expense and the anticipated fewer competitors that possess the capacity to participate in this market.[28] In addition, the definition of value for biologics is more complicated and extends beyond price to include the extent of reimbursement for providers such as health systems and physician offices as well as rebates for pharmacy benefit managers and payers.[12] In order to obtain market share, biosimilar manufacturers will have to define both a price and a reimbursement threshold that is attractive to different audiences.[12] Furthermore, while prices will be lower, the patient cost exposure could remain high, necessitating high-value, accessible patient assistance programs to accompany the launch of biosimilars.

The limited understanding of this new category of medications, the variable and ongoing interpretation of critical regulatory and legal standards, and an extremely complicated definition of perceived financial value combine to create an environment resistant to clarity and difficult to embrace.[17,28] As with other areas in healthcare that are complicated and challenging to define, the need for pharmacist intervention and leadership is exceedingly clear.

THE ESSENTIAL ROLE OF HEALTH-SYSTEM PHARMACISTS IN SUPPORTING THE BIOSIMILAR PARADIGM

Although all clinicians must better understand the principles of biosimilarity, as primary stewards of drug information, providers of patient medication education, and forecasters of pharmaceutical expenditures, pharmacists must possess a complete and objective perspective to support the appropriate evaluation, adoption, and use of these agents. Developing the depth of knowledge required to fulfill this role will not be easy and will necessitate continued attention and repetition. This degree of commitment is absolutely essential to sustain a biosimilars market that delivers on the promise of cost savings. Pharmacists must understand not only the regulatory requirements for biosimilars, but need to increase their familiarity with FDA approval processes as a whole. In addition, they will need to appreciate a multitude of market factors that influence pharmaceutical uptake and success including pricing strategies, managed care influences, expert organization recommendations, advocacy group pressures, and legal determinations. Finally, pharmacists will have to establish review processes sophisticated enough to discern the value of a biosimilar as compared to an originator biologic in terms of price, reimbursement, and patient assistance.

KEY POINTS

- While now very successful, the generic drug experience did not find immediate acceptance. These challenges should inform our expectations for the biosimilar environment.

- Much of the infrastructure that has been established to manage generic drugs as well as high cost originators, both small molecule and biologic, can be used to support the adoption of biosimilars.

CONCLUSION

The introduction of biosimilars comes at a unique time in healthcare where the cost of novel medications is so great, the ability to maintain patient access to needed therapies is imperiled. A successful biosimilars market is critical to any hopes of altering the growth rate of pharmaceutical expenditures and bringing additional calm and stability to a supply chain that is increasingly fragile. The generic experience offers some insight into the degree of financial impact that is possible, although the increased complexity of the healthcare landscape prevents a direct correlation. Conversely, the degree of pharmacists' intervention and advocacy will directly correlate with the extent of success for biosimilars.

REFERENCES

1. Schwartz LL. The debate over substitution policy. Its evolution and scientific basis. *Am J Med.* 1985; 79(suppl 2B):38-44.
2. Generic Pharmaceutical Association. GPhA 2016 generic drug savings and access report. www.gphaonline.org/media/generic-drug-savings-2016/index.html (accessed 3 Oct 2017).
3. Thayer AM. 30 years of generics. *Chem Eng News.* 2014; 92:8-16.
4. Lamy PP. Generic equivalents: issues and concerns. *J Clin Pharmacol.* 1986;26:309-16.
5. Strom BL. Generic drug substitution revisited. *N Engl J Med.* 1987; 316:1456-62.
6. Asclone FJ, Kirking DM, Gaither CA, Welage LS. Historical overview of generic medication policy. *J Am Pharm Assoc.* 2001; 41:567-77.
7. Hamrell MR, Martinez MN, Shrikant VD, Parkman PD. Bioequivalence of generic thioridazine drug products—the FDA viewpoint. *Drug Intell Clin Pharm.* 1987; 21:362-72.
8. Boehm G, Yao Lixin, Han Liang, Zheng Q. Development of the generic drug industry in the US after the Hatch-Waxman Act of 1984. *Acta Pharmaceutica Sinica B.* 2013; 3:297-311.
9. Gibson RM, Waldo DR. National health expenditures, 1980. *Health Care Financ Rev.* 1981; 3:1-54.
10. QuintilesIMS. Medicines use and spending in the U.S. A review of 2016 and outlook to 2021. www.imshealth.com/en/thought-leadership/quintilesims-institute/reports/medicines-use-and-spending-in-the-us-review-of-2016-outlook-to-2021 (accessed 3 Oct 2017).
11. Edwards HS. When the price of the blood pressure drug Nitropress leaped from $215 to $881 last year, an increase of 310%, it triggered public outrage: What's behind the gouging? *Time.* 2016 (May 5); 187(20):38-43.
12. Mulcahy AW, Predmore Z, Mattke S. The cost savings potential of biosimilar drugs in the United States. https://www.rand.org/content/dam/rand/pubs/perspectives/PE100/PE127/RAND_PE127.pdf (accessed 3 Oct 2017).
13. Patel BN, Audet PR. A review of approaches for the management of specialty pharmaceuticals in the United States. *Pharmacoeconomics.* 2014; 32:1105-14.
14. CVS Health. 2017 Standard formulary list of removals and updates. http://investors.cvshealth.com/~/media/Files/C/CVS-IR-v3/documents/02-aug-2016/2017-standard-formulary-list-of-removals-and-updates.pdf (accessed 3 Oct 2017).
15. Lucio SD, Stevenson JG, Hoffman JM. Biosimilars: implications for health-system pharmacists. *Am J Health Syst Pharm.* 2013; 70:2004-2017.
16. Biosimilars approved in Europe. GABI online. http://www.gabionline.net/Biosimilars/General/Biosimilars-approved-in-Europe (accessed 3 Oct 2017).
17. Weise M, Bielsky MC, De Smet K et al. Biosimilars: what clinicians should know. *Blood.* 2012; 120:5111-7.

18. Delivering on the potential of biosimilar medicines: the role of functioning competitive markets. IMS Health, March 2016. www.imshealth.com/files/web/IMSH%20Institute/Healthcare%20Briefs/Documents/IMS_Institute_Biosimilar_Brief_March_2016.pdf (accessed 3 Oct 2017).

19. Grabowski H, Guha R, Salgado M. Biosimilar competition: lessons from Europe. *Nat Rev Drug Discov*. 2014; 13:99-100. Supplementary information.

20. Holmes DR Jr, Becker JA, Granger CB et al. ACCF/AHA 2011 health policy statement on therapeutic interchange and substitution: a report of the American College of Cardiology Foundation Clinical Quality Committee. *J Am Coll Cardiol*. 2011; 58:1287-307.

21. Food and Drug Administration. Guidance for industry, draft guidance. Considerations in demonstrating interchangeability with a reference product. www.fda.gov/downloads/Drugs/GuidanceComplianceRegulatoryInformation/Guidances/UCM537135.pdf (accessed 3 Oct 2017).

22. Food and Drug Administration. Guidance for industry. Biosimilars: questions and answers regarding implementation of the Biologics Price Competition and Innovation Act of 2009, final guidance, April 2015. www.fda.gov/downloads/drugs/guidancecomplianceregulatoryinformation/guidances/ucm444661.pdf (accessed 3 Oct 2017).

23. Cauchi R. State laws and legislation related to biologic medications and substitution of biosimilars. www.ncsl.org/research/health/state-laws-and-legislation-related-to-biologic-medications-and-substitution-of-biosimilars.aspx (accessed 3 Oct 2017).

24. Food and Drug Administration. Guidance for industry. Nonproprietary naming of biological products, draft guidance, August 2015. www.fda.gov/downloads/drugs/guidancecomplianceregulatoryinformation/guidances/ucm459987.pdf (accessed 3 Oct 2017).

25. Kessleheim AS, Woloshin S, Eddings W et al. Physician's knowledge about FDA approval standards and perceptions of the "Breakthrough Therapy" designation. *JAMA*. 2016; 315:1516-8.

26. Kesselheim AS, Eddings W, Raj T et al. Physicians' trust in the FDA's use of product-specific pathways for generic drug approval. *PloS One*. 2016; 11:1-14.

27. Sanchez CK, Zurek AM. Patient perceptions of generic drugs: dispelling misconceptions. *US Pharm*. 2016; 41(generic drugs suppl):36-41.

28. Grabowski HG, Guha R, Salgado M. Regulatory and cost barriers are likely to limit biosimilar development and expected savings in the near future. *Health Aff (Millwood)*. 2014; 33:1048-57.

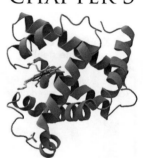

CHAPTER 3

BUGS AND DRUGS, AND YEAST AND MICE, AND CHINESE HAMSTERS

To understand the biosimilar concept, we must ensure adequate familiarity with its associated terminology. *Biosimilars* are highly comparable versions of previously approved biologics. However, the regulatory definition of a biologic is quite broad covering a range of products including a "virus, therapeutic serum, toxin, antitoxin, blood, blood component or derivative, allergenic product, or analogous product, . . . applicable to the prevention, treatment, or cure of a disease or condition of human beings."[1] The biologic definition also includes "therapeutic proteins derived from plants, animals, humans, or microorganisms, and recombinant versions of these products."[1] We should focus our attention on the last part of the definition as the biosimilars currently under development are versions of previously approved, recombinant, originator biologics.[2] A fundamental appreciation of recombinant biologic manufacturing and its associated challenges is essential to improving our vision of the biosimilars market.

The era of recombinant derived biologic drugs officially began with the approval of human insulin in 1982.[3] Since then, pharmaceutical manufacturers have continued to harness the capabilities of recombinant DNA (rDNA) to introduce an ever-increasing number of novel biologics such that the concept of innovation has become synonymous with the success of the biotechnology industry. Although the prospect of developing a replica of a preexisting biologic entity may seem like a more modest technological achievement, it is in fact quite an accomplishment of reverse engineering and requires substantial expertise and manufacturing capabilities.[3] In this chapter, we will examine how advances in biologic manufacturing and regulatory recognition of those innovations have opened the door to both enhancements of originator products as well as the development of biosimilars.[3]

INTRODUCTION TO BIOLOGIC MANUFACTURING

Understanding the Recombinant Manufacturing Process

Recombinant biological manufacturing is a complex endeavor that requires management of a multitude of production-related variables, any of which can impact the final quality, and by extension, safety and efficacy of a biologic pharmaceutical.[3,4] **Figure 3-1** illustrates at a high level the major steps of rDNA development of biologic pharmaceuticals including cell line creation and expansion, protein isolation and purification, and, ultimately, formulation and drug product packaging for patient use.[4] Each step in this process must be closely monitored and well-controlled to minimize any variation that could ultimately compromise the clinical performance of the end product.

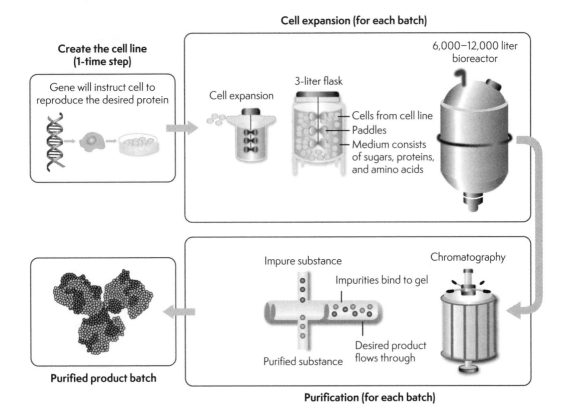

Create the cell line (1-time step)

Gene will instruct cell to reproduce the desired protein

Cell expansion (for each batch)

Cell expansion

3-liter flask

— Cells from cell line
— Paddles
— Medium consists of sugars, proteins, and amino acids

6,000–12,000 liter bioreactor

Impure substance

Impurities bind to gel

Chromatography

Desired product flows through

Purified substance

Purified product batch

Purification (for each batch)

FIGURE 3-1. OVERVIEW OF RECOMBINANT MANUFACTURING PROCESS.

Source: Reprinted from: Al-Sabbagh A, Olech E, McClellan JE, Kirchhoff CF. Development of biosimilars. *Semin Arthritis Rheum.* 2016; 45:S11-8. With permission of Elsevier.

Unlike the chemical synthesis of small molecule medications, the development of a biologic pharmaceutical through rDNA manufacturing begins with the integration of a gene sequence into a living organism, or expression system.[4] These genetically-modified host cells, frequently bacterial, yeast, or mammalian in origin, produce a desired therapeutic protein with the necessary amino acid sequence, higher-order structure, and if required, appropriate post-translational modifications (PTMs), such as glycosylation—all of which contribute to a biologic's desired structure and function.[5]

A great deal of effort is focused on keeping these cell expression systems viable, growing optimally, and free of any contamination.[6] Any change in the cell environment such as the pH, temperature, oxygenation levels, and nutrients, can alter the resulting biologic product.[6] Cell expression systems must be protected from exposure to and contamination by other microorganisms including bacteria, fungi, and viruses.[6] Desired cell expression systems are those that can remain viable under closely managed conditions.[6]

Over the course of the biotechnology era, certain expression systems have come into more routine use given their demonstrated safety, ease of modification, and reliability. As seen in **Table 3-1**, two systems are used quite commonly across frequently prescribed biologics, *Escherichia coli* (*E. coli*) bacteria and Chinese hamster ovary (CHO) cells.[5,7-9]

TABLE 3-1. Expression Systems for Commonly Used Biologic Drugs[5,7-9]		
Drug Name	**Expression System**	**FDA Regulatory Classification**
Adalimumab	CHO	Biologic
Bevacizumab	CHO	Biologic
Cetuximab	Sp2/0	Biologic
Darbepoetin	CHO	Biologic
Epoetin	CHO	Biologic
Etanercept	CHO	Biologic
Filgrastim	*E. coli*	Biologic
Glucagon	*E. coli*	Drug*
Infliximab	Sp2/0	Biologic
Insulin (regular)	*E. coli*	Drug*
Insulin (glargine)	*E. coli*	Drug*
Pegfilgrastim	*E. coli*	Biologic
Rituximab	CHO	Biologic
Somatropin	*E. coli*	Drug*
Trastuzumab	CHO	Biologic

*As of March 23, 2020, certain recombinant products that previously were regulated as drugs will now be regulated as biologics, per the provisions of the Biologics Price Competition and Innovation Act of 2009.[10]

CHO = Chinese hamster ovary; *E. coli* = *Escherichia coli*; Sp2/0 = murine myeloma cells.

Manufacturing Success with Gut Bacteria and Chinese Hamsters

Escherichia coli

The first expression platform used in the biotechnology era was *E. coli*.[5] This expression system has frequently been used in the development and production of biologic products such as insulin and human growth hormone (somatropin), smaller protein therapeutics that do not possess complex PTMs.[5] *E. coli* is a relatively inexpensive system that has demonstrated the reliability needed for pharmaceutical manufacturing, has relatively simple cultivation requirements, and a short generation time.[5] However, this system is not of use when PTMs are essential to the function of a desired protein. For the more complicated biologics such as monoclonal antibodies where PTMs are essential for clinical effect, other cell lines, such as mouse myeloma cells (including NS0 and Sp2/0) and the previously mentioned CHO cells are used.[11] It should also be noted that proteins expressed from *E. coli* systems are produced in an inactive, insoluble form as inclusion bodies, which can make recovery more challenging.[5]

Chinese Hamster Ovary Cells

The cells of a rodent from the deserts of northern China and Mongolia may sound like a rather exotic choice for a prominent component of recombinant biotechnology. However, Chinese hamsters have played a role in the laboratory setting dating back to 1919 when they were used in place of mice for typing pneumococci.[12] Their utility in biologic manufacturing relates to several characteristics that make them particularly useful in the industrial setting. First, CHO cells easily accept genetic modification and the introduction of foreign DNA.[12] They produce the desired biological, with required PTMs, at maximum attainable yields and prevent the introduction and/or propagation of any pathogenic agent that would ultimately be administered to humans.[12] CHO cells also can adapt to growth in a suspension instead of an adherent culture, which allows for increased scale and the use of large, stirred-tank bioreactors.[12] Finally, CHO cells secrete recombinant proteins into media in a natural form.[12]

Protein Growth, Isolation, Purification, Formulation, and Drug Packaging

As described above, the choice of cell expression system and development of the specific cell line creates additional considerations in relation to protein extraction given the environment and form in which the recombinant product is secreted.[5] Even beyond the expression system, the processes occurring during the extraction and purification of proteins can damage the biologic through oxidation, reduction, deamidation, and fragmentation.[13] These steps can also result in protein aggregation and/or the introduction of process-related impurities.[13] As a result, manufacturers must closely monitor the components of product purification including the choice of detergent or solvent for extraction, the filtration system and column material used, the input protein concentration, pH, solvent system, and ionic strength and charge for the final purification steps.[13]

MANAGING BIOLOGIC VARIATION

The Product Is the Process ...or Is It?

The expression systems previously described can and have been used very successfully to produce biologic products. However, these living organisms also introduce variation in the complex biologics they create.[3] Unlike chemical mechanisms where identical molecules can be replicated continuously, living organisms do not produce exact copies of a biologic throughout each cycle of growth.[3] As compared to the molecular structures of small molecules, biologics are much larger and more complicated, resulting in the opportunity for variation across a vast array of product attributes.[3] The production of biological medications involves the continual refinement of manufacturing processes.[3] Any modification in the conditions under which cells are managed can affect the functioning of the expression system and by extension, the biologic products that are produced.[3] Biologic manufacturing necessitates a continuous oversight of the totality of process steps to ensure a tight control of all quality attributes that influence the molecule's clinical functioning.[4] Failure to manage unintended or unexpected changes in a biologic's key quality parameters, known as drift, could result in negative clinical outcomes.[14]

This intrinsic interrelationship of the manufacturing steps with the activity of the resulting biologic product has historically been characterized by phrases such as "the product is the process," meaning that a modification to any of the production activities will inherently result in a different biologic.[15] This paradigm would seem to represent an immovable barrier to the development of a biosimilar since the proprietary and confidential nature of the originator molecule's manufacturing process cannot be exactly replicated by the biosimilar applicant.[3] Instead, biosimilar manufacturers must use unique production processes, including different expression system cell cultures to create their related biologics.[3] Fortunately, originator manufacturers and regulatory authorities encountered this problem long before the advent of biosimilars. As a result, regulations coupled with analytical advancements have now enabled the biologics market to overcome the "product is the process" barrier.[16]

Snowflakes, Diamonds, and the Principle of Comparability

A frequent visual and verbal metaphor used to describe biologic variation is the example of snowflakes.[17] Just as we characterize no two snowflakes as having identical structures, the differences between originator biologics and biosimilars are frequently illustrated via the example in **Figure 3-2**:

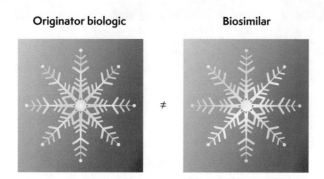

Originator biologic   Biosimilar

$\neq$

FIGURE 3-2. TRADITIONAL ILLUSTRATION OF ORIGINATOR BIOLOGICS AND BIOSIMILARS.

Given the size and complexity of biologic molecules, coupled with differences in their manufacturing, this description is true, to a point.[3,17] Originator biologics and biosimilars are not identical products.[3] Therefore, any characterization as generic, which would imply an exact copy, would be inaccurate.[6] However, there is more detail to this visual story. Just as biosimilars differ from the originator biologic, so does the originator differ from itself over the course of its life cycle.[16]

An originator reference biologic is not a static entity.[3,16] In addition to the inherent variability that is a byproduct of recombinant manufacturing, additional variations arise as process changes are introduced to increase scale, produce greater product yields, improve product purity, create new formulations of the originator biologic, or even relocate production.[3,15,16] Each of these changes introduces modifications that while well controlled and monitored, result in a slightly different version of the originator molecule.[3,16] Following such a manufacturing modification, a post-change version of the originator biologic, while similar, is not identical to its pre-change version as shown in **Figure 3-3**.[3,16]

Still, this representation fails to capture the full aspect of the highly similar, but variable nature of biologic formulations. As marketed biologics are collections of similar molecules, a more appropriate view of biologics would be as mixtures of snowflakes, or diamonds as shown in the **Figure 3-4**, another naturally occurring (and more expensive) substance for which no two examples are considered identical.[16,18] Originator biologics demonstrate variability from batch to batch and from lot to lot.[3,16] Additional variation is introduced when manufacturing changes are made to branded biologics.[3,16] Biosimilars, which are derived from different manufacturing

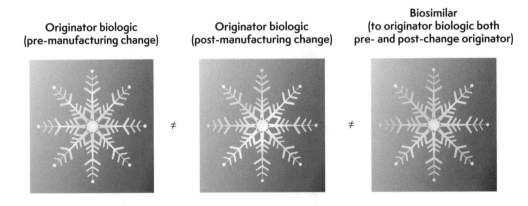

FIGURE 3-3. EXPANDED ILLUSTRATION OF ORIGINATOR BIOLOGICS (INCLUDING MODIFICATIONS) AND BIOSIMILARS.

processes will also vary.[3,16] However, regulatory standards for originator changes, known as comparability, have been in place for 20 years to ensure these variations, while present, do not contribute to meaningful differences in clinical safety or efficacy.[3,16] In order to understand biosimilarity, we must first appreciate the comparability standard.

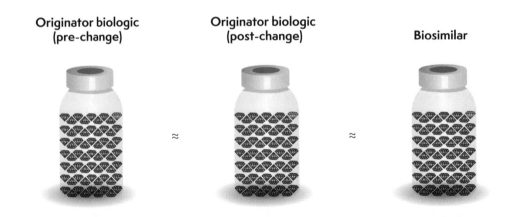

FIGURE 3-4. ENHANCED ILLUSTRATION, ORIGINATOR BIOLOGIC AND BIOSIMILAR VARIABILITY.[16,18]

Before Biosimilarity, There Was Comparability

To allow product enhancement and related manufacturing changes, yet maintain a consistency throughout the life cycle of an originator biologic, an additional regulatory approach to evaluate similarity before and after a manufacturing change was required. In 1996, the U.S. Food and Drug Administration (FDA) took the global regulatory lead in defining the concept of comparability in its guidance document, "Demonstration of Comparability of Human Biological Products."[19] This regulation articulated an approach by which manufacturing changes could be made so that the resulting variability of a biologic would remain within a narrow range allowing a product, post-manufacturing change to be considered equivalent, or "comparable" to the pre-manu-facturing change version.[16] In addition, this standard recognized that analytical characterization of a manufacturing change might be sufficient such that additional clinical studies to evaluate product safety and efficacy of the post-change product might not be required.[16]

In 2005, the International Conference on Harmonization (ICH), an international body that works to establish commonality for pharmaceutical evaluation across the highly regulated markets of the United States, the European Union (EU), and Japan incorporated this approach into its standards.[16] This document, known as ICH Q5E, "Comparability of Biotechnological/ Biological Products Subject to Changes in their Manufacturing Process," has helped direct the validation of the safety and efficacy of manufacturing changes to originator reference mole-cules.[20] This capability has been critically important to the pharmaceutical industry given that manufacturing changes have occurred across many of the biologics commonly prescribed in markets such as the EU and the United States.[21] **Table 3-2** lists manufacturing changes for commonly used biologics, the monoclonal antibodies, as identified through the publicly avail-able European Public Assessment Report documents.[22]

The degree of risk associated with various changes can be stratified (**Table 3-3**). Although many changes are considered low risk, a reasonable number involve some degree of change to the active substance or a starting material, reagent, or intermediate substance.[22] In spite of the complexity and importance of these changes, the principles of comparability have enabled those modifications to occur while validating that the pre- and post-change products do not differ in terms of safety, purity, and potency.[16] In addition, the post-change product retains the same branded name, nonproprietary name, and labeling as the pre-change version.[16] Most changes

TABLE 3-2. Manufacturing Changes for Monoclonal Antibodies per European Public Assessment Reports[a,22]

Drug	Number of Changes with Low Risk	Number of Changes with Moderate Risk	Number of Changes with High Risk	Total Changes	Average Change Per Product Year
Rituximab	7	15	1	23	1.44
Palivizumab	1	16	1	18	1.20
Infliximab	13	34	3	50	3.33
Trastuzumab	1	23	2	26	1.86
Adalimumab	8	17	3	28	2.55
Cetuximab	3	17	0	20	2.00
Bevacizumab	4	8	0	12	1.33
Panitumumab	1	10	0	11	1.57
Certolizumab pegol	2	13	0	15	3.00
Golimumab	3	8	2	13	2.60
Tocilizumab	2	4	1	7	1.40
Ipilimumab	3	8	0	11	3.67

[a]Products approved by European Medicines Agency 1998—October 2014.

TABLE 3-3. Description of Manufacturing Change Types[22]

Type of Manufacturing Change	Description
Low risk	■ Change associated with the finished product (FP) including replacement or addition of manufacturing site, modification of in-process tests or limits, difference in immediate packaging, or changes to production facility
Moderate risk	■ Change(s) to the manufacturing process of the active substance (AS) such as change in manufacturer of AS or starting material/reagent/intermediate, modification of in-process tests or limits of the AS
High risk	■ Change in the purification of the AS or in the synthesis or recovery of a nonpharmacopoeial or novel excipient ■ Change in the manufacturer of AS or of a starting material/reagent/intermediate for AS ■ Change in AS or intermediate batch size (including batch size ranges) ■ Change to in-process tests or limits applied during the manufacture of AS, such as widening of the approved in-process test limits (which could significantly affect the overall quality of the AS)

are approved without the need for additional clinical studies and all of these changes proceed without the awareness of prescriber or patient communities that a modification has occurred.[16]

Manufacturing-related change information is not made publicly accessible for U.S. licensed biologics. However, the similarity of the U.S. and European markets along with direct comparisons of branded products from both settings suggest a comparable number of manufacturing changes occur for FDA-approved biologic agents.[23-25]

Beyond "The Product Is the Process"

Given the introduction and success of the comparability standard, we can conclude that a highly similar biologic, can be manufactured even if its production steps have been modified.[16,21,22] Consequently, a biologic product is no longer inextricably tied to its manufacturing steps.[16,21] The comparability standard served as the template upon which the European approach to biosimilars was established.[16] In addition, FDA in its advisory guidance on biosimilars notes the concepts shared between biosimilarity and comparability. However, FDA also states that the data requirement for biosimilarity will be greater because the originator company has complete oversight of their manufacturing processes, including life cycle changes.[26] Still, as with comparability, much of the additional information required for a biosimilar application will be in the form of analytical characterization data.[26] As we continue to proceed into this new era of biologic competition, we must remain cognizant of the fact that many of the basic concepts for ensuring the safety of manufacturing changes long have predated the advent of biosimilars.

THE IMPORTANCE OF HIGH QUALITY MANUFACTURING FOR ALL PHARMACEUTICALS

As we have seen in this chapter, the quality of biologic manufacturing is directly correlated with the safety and efficacy profile of the resulting medication, originator or biosimilar.[3,4] As such, this aspect of manufacturing will remain critical for initial product launches, comparability determinations, and biosimilarity reviews.[3,4,16] A recent example of the impact of biologic manufacturing quality on product licensing was demonstrated with the approval efforts for biosimilar epoetin alfa (Epogen®; Amgen).[27] Pfizer has continued in its efforts to receive licensing for a biosimilar epoetin and has even progressed to the point where an FDA advisory committee overwhelmingly recommended approval of their product.[27] However, the FDA ultimately issued a complete response letter delaying final endorsement due to previously identified manufacturing issues at the location the biosimilar was possibly going to be produced.[28]

Also, this focus on biologic manufacturing should elevate our awareness regarding the quality issues we have seen with the production of small molecule medications. While we are opening a new frontier of biologic competition, the generic market is continuing down an almost two decade's long path of drug shortages, supply interruptions, and recalls primarily due to manufacturing problems.[29] Hopefully, the greater degree of investment in biologic manufacturing and the new production capabilities will insulate biosimilars from this issue. Still, we should use the increased scrutiny of biologic and biosimilar development to increase our collective understanding of the essential relationship between quality manufacturing and a robust and stable supply of all molecules.

KEY POINTS

- Recombinant DNA technology is the essential element of biologic manufacturing and supports the development of high quality, yet variable products.

- Even prior to biosimilarity, comparability provisions were established to ensure manufacturing changes did not affect the safety and efficacy of modified biologics.

- The comparability principle, which allows for the safe modification of originator biologics, is closely related to the biosimilar paradigm that supports the licensing of highly similar versions of biologics (i.e., biosimilars). Given the extended history of safety and success, the similarity of these processes should improve our confidence in the manufacturing of biosimilars.

CONCLUSION

The recombinant biologic manufacturing process is very complex and highly sensitive to any change. Any attempts to create a highly similar version of a preexisting biologic require a substantial level of skill and expertise to manage the variables that could create undesirable variations. However, the concept of highly similar biologic drugs developed through different manufacturing steps is not novel to the biosimilars' experience, but has been an essential and well-vetted component of originator biologic production. The increased knowledge associated with several decades of originator biotechnology success coupled with the experience of biosimilar development in Europe has provided a foundation on which the U.S. biosimilar market can be constructed.

REFERENCES

1. Food and Drug Administration. Frequently asked questions about therapeutic biological products. www.fda.gov/Drugs/DevelopmentApprovalProcess/HowDrugsareDevelopedandApproved/ApprovalApplications/TherapeuticBiologicApplications/ucm113522.htm. (accessed 3 Oct. 2017).
2. IMS Health. Medicines use and spending shifts in the U.S.—a review of 2015 and outlook to 2020, April 2016. www.imshealth.com/en/thought-leadership/quintilesims-institute/reports/medicines-use-and-spending-in-the-us-a-review-of-2015-and-outlook-to-2020 (accessed 3 Oct. 2017).
3. Tsuruta LR, Lopes dos Santos M, Moro AM. Biosimilars advancements: moving on to the future. *Biotechnol Prog.* 2015; 31:1139-49.
4. Al-Sabbagh A, Olech E, McClellan JE, Kirchhoff CF. Development of biosimilars. *Semin Arthritis Rheum.* 2016; 45:S11-8.
5. Dingermann T. Recombinant therapeutic proteins: production platforms and challenges. *Biotechnol J.* 2008; 3:90-7.
6. Geigert J. Biologics are not chemical drugs. In: *The Challenge of CMC Regulatory Compliance for Biopharmaceuticals and Other Biologics.* New York: Springer, 2013.
7. Reichert JM. Marketed therapeutic antibodies compendium. *mAbs.* 2012; 4:413-5.
8. Jelkmann W. Recombinant EPO production—points the nephrologist should know. *Nephrol Dial Transplant.* 2007; 22:2749-53.
9. Egrie JC, Dwyer E, Browne JK, Lykos MA. Darbepoetin alfa has a longer circulating half-life and greater in vivo potency than recombinant human erythropoietin. *Exp Hematol.* 2003; 31:290-9.
10. Title VII: Improving access to innovative medical therapies. Subtitle A: Biologic Price Competition and Innovation provisions of the Patient Protection and Affordable Care Act (PPACA). www.fda.gov/downloads/Drugs/GuidanceComplianceRegulatoryInformation/ucm216146.pdf (accessed 3 Oct. 2017).
11. Kantardjieff A, Zhou W. Mammalian cell cultures for biologics manufacturing. *Adv Biochem Eng Biotechnol.* 2014; 139:1-9.
12. Jayapal KP, Wlaschin KF, Hu WS, Yap MGS. Recombinant protein therapeutics from CHO cells—20 years and counting. CHO Consortium, SBE Special Edition. www.aiche.org/sites/default/files/docs/pages/CHO.pdf. (accessed 3 Oct. 2017).
13. Ahmed I, Kaspar B, Sharma U. Biosimilars: impact of biologic product life cycle and European experience on the regulatory trajectory in the United States. *Clin Ther.* 2012; 34:400-19.
14. Bui LA, Hurst A, Finch GL et al. Key considerations in the preclinical development of biosimilars. *Drug Discov Today.* 2015; 20(suppl 1):3-15.

15. Tsiftsoglou AS, Trouvin JH, Calvo G, Ruiz S. Demonstration of biosimilarity, extrapolation of indications and other challenges related to biosimilars in Europe. *BioDrugs* 2014; 28:479-86.

16. McCamish M, Woollett G. Worldwide experience with biosimilar development. *mAbs* 2011; 3:209-17.

17. Lorenzetti L. Biosimilars may one day save your live. But what are they? http://fortune.com/2015/02/06/biosimilars-what-are-they/ (accessed 3 Oct. 2017).

18. Diamond Quality Factors, Gemological Institute of America. www.gia.edu/diamond-quality-factor (accessed 3 Oct. 2017).

19. FDA. Demonstration of comparability of human biological products, including therapeutic biotechnology-derived products. www.fda.gov/Drugs/GuidanceComplianceRegulatoryInformation/Guidances/ucm122879.htm (accessed 3 Oct. 2017).

20. FDA. ICH Q5E: Comparability of biotechnological/biological products subject to changes in their manufacturing process. www.fda.gov/OHRMS/DOCKETS/98fr/2004d-0118-gdl0001.pdf (accessed 3 Oct. 2017).

21. Schiestl M, Stangler T, Torell C, et al. Acceptable changes in quality attributes of glycosylated biopharmaceuticals. *Nat Biotechnol.* 2011; 29:310-2.

22. Vezer B, Buzas Z, Sebeszta M, Zrubka Z. Authorized manufacturing changes for therapeutic monoclonal antibodies (mAbs) in European Public Assessment Report (EPAR) documents. *Curr Med Res Opin.* 2016; 32:829-34.

23. FDA briefing document. BLA 125544, CT-P13, a proposed biosimilar to Remicade (infliximab). Arthritis Advisory Committee Meeting. February 9, 2016. www.fda.gov/downloads/AdvisoryCommittees/CommitteesMeetingMaterials/Drugs/ArthritisAdvisoryCommittee/UCM484859.pdf (accessed Oct. 3, 2017).

24. FDA briefing document. BLA 761024, ABP 501, a proposed biosimilar to Humira (adalimumab). Arthritis Advisory Committee Meeting. July 12, 2016. www.fda.gov/downloads/AdvisoryCommittees/CommitteesMeetingMaterials/Drugs/ArthritisAdvisoryCommittee/UCM510293.pdf (accessed Oct. 3, 2017).

25. FDA briefing document. BLA 761042, GP2015, a proposed biosimilar to Enbrel (etanercept). Arthritis Advisory Committee Meeting. July 13, 2016. www.fda.gov/downloads/AdvisoryCommittees/CommitteesMeetingMaterials/Drugs/ArthritisAdvisoryCommittee/UCM510493.pdf (accessed Oct. 3, 2017).

26. Food and Drug Administration. Guidance for industry. Scientific considerations in demonstrating biosimilarity to a reference product, April 2015. www.fda.gov/downloads/drugs/guidancecomplianceregulatoryinformation/guidances/ucm291128.pdf (accessed Oct. 3, 2017).

27. Stanton D. Second time the charm for Pfizer's Epogen biosimilar in the US. http://www.biopharma-reporter.com/Markets-Regulations/US-FDA-votes-in-favour-of-Pfizer-s-Epogen-biosimilar (accessed Oct. 3, 2017).

28. Mehr S. FDA stuns with rejection of Pfizer's Retacrit. https://biosimilarsrr.com/2017/06/26/fda-stuns-with-rejection-of-pfizers-retacrit/ (accessed Oct. 3, 2017).

29. Woodcock J, Wosinska M. Economic and technological drivers of generic sterile injectable drug shortages. *Clin Pharmacol Ther.* 2013; 93:170-6.

CHAPTER 4

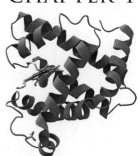

THE $250 BILLION PYRAMID: ANALYTICS IN BIOSIMILARITY DETERMINATION

The foundation of a biosimilarity exercise is the comparative analytical characterization used to establish and confirm that a proposed biosimilar has a comparable structure and function to that of an originator reference product.[1] The application and continued advancement of these techniques are enabling the realization of the U.S. biosimilars market by supporting an approval process where duplicative clinical trial data requirements are minimized, thus allowing for lower development costs and the opportunity for less expensive alternatives to commonly-utilized branded biologics.[2] Two critical challenges must be addressed regarding the role of analytical data in the pharmaceutical supply environment. First, most practitioners, including pharmacists, have limited familiarity with the purpose or meaning of analytical characterization tests, which degrades the extent to which this information provides reassurance of a biosimilar's safety and efficacy.[3] Second, most clinicians by training and routine are conditioned to seek and demand clinical evaluations for pharmaceuticals, particularly those as complex as biologics.[3,4] Therefore, to support a receptive culture to biosimilars, clinicians must have a sound foundational understanding of the analytical tools and techniques that substantiate the similarity of biologicals and their validity in relation to clinical trial data.

IT'S ALL ABOUT THE BASE!

The Food and Drug Administration (FDA) and other authors have described the biosimilar approval process and its relationship to the licensing pathway of originator through the use of triangles or pyramids as shown in Figure 4-1.[5,6] For an originator reference product, the pyramid is inverted meaning the extent of information known about a novel molecule expands through each successive phase of investigation.[5] Conversely, the biosimilar pyramid is oriented in a traditional fashion. At the base of the pyramid is the broader foundation of analytical characterization upon which all subsequent, and more targeted phases, are built.[6] Given that a reference product has been fully characterized by years of review and use, the intent of biosimilar development is first to establish analytical similarity followed by the use of nonclinical and clinical data to address any residual uncertainties.[6] Estimates suggest that biosimilars could deliver anywhere from $13 billion to $250 billion in savings within a decade's time.[7,8] However, savings of any magnitude are not possible in the absence of analytical characterization.

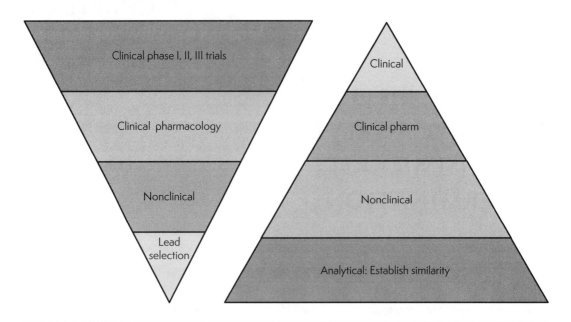

FIGURE 4-1. CONTRASTING THE PYRAMIDS: ORIGINATOR VERSUS BIOSIMILAR APPROVAL.[5]

GOAL POSTS—ESSENTIAL IN BOTH FOOTBALL AND BIOSIMILAR DEVELOPMENT

The development of a biosimilar begins with the identification of the target critical quality attributes (CQAs)—the essential properties of the originator reference product that must be matched.[9] Collectively, these attributes are known as the quality target product profile (QTPP) of the branded biologic or less formally, goal posts.[9,10] This terminology reflects that all biologics demonstrate variability.[10] As described in Chapter 3, it is not a reasonable expectation for each biosimilar to match every characteristic exactly because even the originator fails to meet this level of consistency.[10] Instead, originators vary across a well-defined range, by which the biosimilar must be assessed and matched.[10] To achieve this goal, a biosimilar developer must conduct a detailed evaluation of multiple lots of the originator reference biologic over time to characterize the fluctuation of these attributes and determine the degree of variation.[10] After these properties have been defined, the biosimilar sponsor must then develop a manufacturing process that produces a match of the reference biologic so that the safety and efficacy of the proposed product are preserved.[9,10]

As no single analytical test can sufficiently establish biosimilarity on its own, the task of demonstrating molecular equivalence involves a panel of analytical methods.[11] With the application of currently available advanced technologies, it is now possible to define the molecular similarity between a biosimilar and originator product, even for such complex molecules as monoclonal antibodies.[11] Various sensitive, ultra-high-resolution analytical techniques and robust functional assays have been developed in recent years that allow for a more in-depth characterization of complex proteins to determine similarity in key structural and functional quality attributes between a biosimilar candidate and its reference product.[11,12]

FDA'S PERSPECTIVE ON BIOSIMILAR ANALYTICAL CHARACTERIZATION

In February 2012, FDA articulated its guidance regarding the analytical evaluation of a biosimilar. This document, "Quality Considerations in Demonstrating Biosimilarity of a Therapeutic Protein Product to a Reference Product," was published in its final form in April 2015.[13]

The key attributes FDA identified as critical to the analytical assessment of biosimilarity included the following:

- Expression system
- Manufacturing process
- Assessment of physicochemical properties
- Functional activities
- Receptor binding and immunochemical properties
- Impurities
- Reference product and reference standards
- Finished drug product
- Stability

Each of these factors is important in the validation of a highly similar product. For example, beginning with the manufacturing of a recombinant biologic, a biosimilar supplier would not have access to the exact same cell line developed by the originator due to the proprietary nature of expression systems.[12] The biosimilar manufacturer could employ the same type of cell line (e.g., *Escherichia coli*, Chinese hamster ovary cell).[13] Therefore, an analytical evaluation of the expression system is necessary for a biosimilar application. In addition, the applicant must provide a detailed analysis of the manufacturing steps and data to demonstrate adequate control of all processes and critical attributes for the protein.[9,10]

Ultimately, the resulting biosimilar must be rigorously compared to the originator reference biologic for the following attributes:[11]

- Primary structure, amino acid sequence,
- Higher-order structures, including secondary, tertiary, and quaternary structures,
- Protein concentration,
- Post-translational modification, such as glycosylation, as appropriate,
- Microheterogeneity and product-related substances, such as protein deamidation and oxidation.

A Statistical Approach to Analytical Characterization

In September 2017, the FDA published a companion document to its Quality Considerations guidance entitled, "Statistical Approaches to Evaluate Analytical Similarity."[14] This draft guidance provides additional perspective on how appropriate statistical analyses increase the level of confidence in the analytical characterization of a biosimilar as compared to an originator reference biologic. In this guidance, FDA emphasizes the importance of biosimilar applicants developing risk assessment tools for quality attributes depending on each characteristic's potential for impact on clinical performance or its degree of uncertainty. Not only does this risk assessment identify the attributes of greatest interest, it assists in the determination of which statistical analyses should be applied to assess the molecule.[14] Attributes with the highest risk should be assessed according to the standards of equivalence testing. Lower risk attributes can be evaluated through the use of quality ranges. Finally, the lowest risk attributes can be monitored through visual comparisons.[14] The guidance also articulates the minimum number of biosimilar and originator biologic lots (10 each) for inclusion in the analytical characterization.[14]

THE PRINCIPLE OF ORTHOGONALITY ACROSS ANALYTICAL TECHNIQUES

One of the most important concepts to understand within the context of biosimilar development is the principle of orthogonality. In analytical chemistry, tests that are orthogonal are assays that use different chemical or physical mechanisms to measure the same attribute.[15] The application of multiple, orthogonal assays increases the reliability in the assessment of a particular characteristic of a biologic and provides greater confidence in the outcome of these evaluations. An expectation of FDA or any other regulatory body is that applicants will apply orthogonal tests throughout the development of a biosimilar.[10] **Table 4-1** lists some of the common tests that are used to assess different critical attributes.

Primary Structure

The primary structure is the linear sequence of amino acids that make up a biologic.[2] The sequence of amino acids for a biosimilar must match that of the originator reference product as any variations could alter the functioning of the proposed molecule by impacting its safety and efficacy.[10] Therefore, this attribute is critical to the success of a biosimilar development program. This characteristic is also extremely useful in illustrating certain techniques such as mass spectrometry (MS) and liquid chromatography, specifically reverse phase-high pressure liquid chromatography (RP-HPLC).[12,20]

MS is the process of determining the mass of a molecule by measuring its mass-to-charge ratio, represented as (m/z).[1,16,19] Proteins are made up of a sequence of amino acids, subunits that possess a charge in an ionized state. In MS, molecules are ionized and then subjected to electric and/or magnetic fields, which alter or deflect the paths of the molecules based on their mass and charge.[1,16] The extent to which they are deflected can be used to identify and quantify aspects of the molecules, such as the identity of the amino acid sequence and/or the total molecular weight of the protein. MS can be done in a top down fashion, where the intact biologic is subjected to the mass spectrometer; bottom up, where enzymes are first used to digest the protein into smaller units; or middle up, where the product is separated, but not completely fragmented.[1,2,12,23] All of these iterations would likely be useful for biosimilar characterization.

Another key workhorse in evaluating many aspects of biologic attributes is liquid chromatography, a technique used to separate a sample into individual parts based on its interaction with a mobile and solid phase.[33] In liquid chromatography, a liquid mobile phase is passed through a column containing a solid stationary phase.[33] Samples with greater affinity for the mobile phase will pass through the column more rapidly.[33] Those with increased affinity for the solid phase will progress more slowly.[33] HPLC denotes the use of increased pressures to force the solvent

TABLE 4-1. Analytical Tests Used in Biosimilarity Determination[1,2,10-12,16-36]

Attribute	Technologies Applied	Comments

Primary structure	■ Peptide mapping
	■ RP-HPLC-MS
	   ● ESI
	   ● Matrix-MALDI-TOF
		■ The primary structure is the linear sequence of amino acids that make up a protein.
		■ The amino acid sequence is expected to be identical between the biosimilar and the originator reference product
		■ Peptide maps are developed by selectively cleaving the biosimilar into smaller subunits using certain enzymes
		■ Mass spectrometry ionizes proteins and allows for determination of the mass of the protein and its amino acid sequencing
		   ● ESI and MALDI are two mechanisms to apply a charge to the proteins.
		   ● TOF—Detection process that assesses the impact of mass spectrometry on sample
		■ The result of the liquid chromatography separation and mass spectrometry analysis is a peptide map (i.e., fingerprint) of the biosimilar
		■ Sequencing can be done both bottom up (protein is identified after proteolysis from its peptides), middle up (proteolysis to subunits) or top down (the intact protein is subject to analysis).

(continued)

TABLE 4-1. (Continued)

Attribute	Technologies Applied	Comments

Higher order structure	■ CD—Far and near ultraviolet (UV–CD)
	
	■ FTIR
	
	■ NMR
	
	■ DSC
	
	■ X-ray crystallography
	
	■ HDX-MS
	
	■ Ellman's assay (free thiols)
		■ These studies evaluate aspects of the structural confirmation of the molecule including secondary, tertiary, and quaternary structure, as well as other attributes such as the stability of the protein
		
		■ The choice of analytical tool depends on certain characteristics of the molecule as well as fundamental aspects of proteins
		
		   ● Certain proteins (tryptophan, tyrosine, and phenylalanine) possess intrinsic fluorescence, which can be leveraged to allow for protein assessment
		
		■ CD measures differences in a protein's absorption of left-handed versus right-handed polarized light and provides information on the folding state of the protein
		
		   ● *Far UV*—assesses secondary structure such as alpha helices and beta sheets
		
		   ● *Near UV*—assesses tertiary structure, how secondary elements fold on themselves
		
		■ FTIR provides information on the vibrational states of molecules in the protein (e.g., vibrational states of the amide groups in the biosimilar)—reveals if there are differences in higher order structure (protein folding)
		
		■ *NMR*—Based on the spin of nuclei with odd mass numbers in an external magnetic field; used to create a "fingerprint" of the protein
		
		■ Tests assess not only the structure under resting conditions, but under stress (i.e., DSC—identifies point at which molecule begins to change)
		
		■ *X-ray crystallography*—a crystallized protein sample is exposed to an x ray beam that creates a diffraction pattern allowing evaluation of the three-dimensional structure of the biologic
		
		■ *HDX-MS*—Exchange of deuterium for hydrogen increases mass, allowing for visibility through MS; enables identification of changes in the secondary structure of the biologic
		
		■ *Ellman's reagent*—binds to free thiol groups in a protein; the presence of free thiols could be indicative of the failure to form disulfide bonds potentially leading to a conformation change.

Protein concentration	■ Ultraviolet spectroscopy (UV 280)	■ *UV 280*—Amino acids with aromatic rings (tyrosine and tryptophan) absorb ultraviolet light at a wavelength of 280 nm. The measurement of absorption provides a method to assess total protein concentration as well as contaminants.

(continued)

TABLE 4-1. (Continued)

Attribute	Technologies Applied	Comments
Post-translational modifications (e.g., acetylation, carboxylation, glycosylation, methylation, phosphorylation, sulfation)	■ Oligosaccharide map ■ MALDI-TOF MS ■ RP-HPLC-MS	■ *Oligosaccharide map*—similar to peptide mapping, enzymes cleave the glycan residues from the protein allowing for characterization of these subunits through various technologies incorporating MS ■ *MALDI-TOF MS*—see above ■ High pressure liquid chromatography is the application of high pressures to traditional liquid chromatography techniques to separate mixtures of substances based on their molecular structure and composition. This technique is frequently coupled with MS to identify PTMs.
Higher molecular weight/ aggregation	■ SEC ■ AUC ■ *SDS-PAGE or CE -SDS*—aggregation and fragment ■ Western blot (take SDS page gel–membrane–antibody detects the protein of interest) ■ Field flow fractionation	■ *SEC*—analytical method that uses porous particles to separate molecules of different sizes. Molecules that are smaller than the pore size can enter the particles and, therefore, have a longer path and transit time than molecules that are larger. ■ *AUC*—application of a centrifugal field to a sample causes differences in the distribution of units within the sample based on molecular mass and shape ■ *SDS-PAGE SDS*—an ionic detergent that binds to and denatures proteins to make them uniformly negatively charged. Polyacrilamide is a high molecular weight polymer of acrylamide used as a support and separations matrix. When a current is applied to the gel, the molecules move toward the positively charged electrode. Proteins with less mass travel more quickly through the gel matrix allowing separation. ● *CE-SDS*—Capillary counterpart to SDS-PAGE; test conducted in a capillary tube rather than a slab; capillary format enables automation and provides better resolution ■ *Western blot*—immunochemical method for identifying proteins in a complex mixture, proteins separated by electrophoresis are transferred (blotted) from the gel medium to a membrane; the transferred proteins are then detected by their relative binding to labeled antibodies. ■ *Field flow fractionation*—a flow-based separation methodology. Molecules are separated based on their diffusion coefficients. The retention and separation of samples is controlled by an external field perpendicular to the channel flow.

(continued)

TABLE 4-1. (Continued)

Attribute	Technologies Applied	Comments
Purity, charge heterogeneity, other variants	■ CZE ■ IEF or cIEF ■ Ion exchange chromatography ■ RP-HPLC-MS	■ *CZE*—the simplest form of capillary electrophoresis; separation based on differences in charge-to-mass ratio. As charge is applied, components in a sample separate into discrete zones. ■ *IEF*—electrophoretic technique for separation of proteins based on their isoelectric point (pI), the pH at which the protein has no net charge and does not migrate further in an electric field ■ *Ion exchange chromatography*—separation technique that differentiates samples based on the overall charge of a protein

AUC = analytical ultracentrifugation; CD = circular dichroism; CE-SDS = capillary sodium dodecyl sulfate gel electrophoresis; cIEF = capillary isoelectric focusing; CZE = capillary zone electrophoresis; DSC = differential scanning calorimetry; ESI = electrospray ionization; FTIR = Fourier-transform infrared spectroscopy; HDX-MS = hydrogen/deuterium exchange; IEF = isoelectric focusing; MALDI-TOF= matrix-assisted laser desorption ionization-time of flight; NMR = nuclear magnetic resonance; PTM= post-translational modification; RP-HPLC-MS = reversed phase-high pressure liquid chromatography-mass spectrometry detection; SDS-PAGE = sodium dodecyl sulfate polyacrylamide gel electrophoresis; SEC = size exclusion chromatography.

through the solid phase.[33] In normal phase- high pressure liquid chromatography (NP-HPLC), the stationary phase is polar.[33] Therefore, less polar components will pass through the column more quickly due to fewer interactions with the stationary phase. In RP-HPLC, the polarities of the mobile and stationary phases are reversed (i.e., mobile phase more polar, stationary phase less polar).[35] As a result, more polar components elute first followed by less polar products. As shown in **Figure 4-2**, a peptide mixture is separated via HPLC, after which the units are ionized and directed to a mass spectrometer for further analysis.[38,39]

The use of tools like HPLC and MS allows for the complete and accurate confirmation of an amino acid sequence for a biosimilar.[16] As described below, these tools can also be used to evaluate post-translational modifications (PTMs), such as glycosylation profiles.[16]

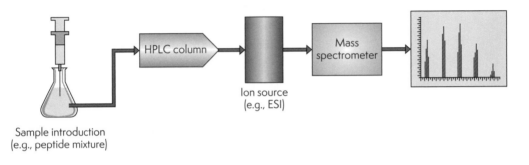

Sample introduction (e.g., peptide mixture)

Ion source (e.g., ESI)

FIGURE 4-2. SIMPLIFIED LIQUID CHROMATOGRAPHY/MASS SPECTROMETRY PROCESS.[37,38]

The accurate sequencing of amino acids is critical to the appropriate functioning of biologics.[13] However, the biosimilars era has not only increased our awareness of this importance, but also emphasized how little attention clinicians have historically paid to these attributes. For example, analytical characterizations of biosimilars have revealed errors in the amino acid sequences of originator biologics (e.g., rituximab and cetuximab) published in public databases.[39] These errors, while having no negative effects on the products, nevertheless, highlight the increasing scrutiny and importance of this attribute now that multiple manufacturers will be supplying versions of the same molecule. A tangential benefit of biosimilars will be the increased awareness and understanding of the potential variability of all biologics and the extent to which such changes are monitored.

Higher Order Structure

In addition to an identical amino acid sequence, biosimilars must possess a higher order structure that is comparable to the originator reference product. Higher order structures are classified as secondary, tertiary, quaternary, all of which must be thoroughly vetted within a biosimilarity exercise.[2] Secondary structures refer to regular, structural units such as right-handed, helical-coiled strands, called α-helices, or stretched, peptide chains, called β-sheets.[2] The interaction between these secondary elements to form the three-dimensional shape of a biologic protein is called the tertiary structure.[2] Finally, many proteins are made up of multiple polypeptide chains, often called protein subunits. The quaternary structure is defined by the way these protein subunits interact with each other and arrange themselves to form a larger aggregate protein complex.[2] **Figure 4-3** illustrates the relationship of these various layers of biologic structure.[40,41]

As listed in Table 4-1 above, many tests are available to assess higher order structure. Commonly used techniques include circular dichroism (CD), Fourier transform infrared spectroscopy (FTIR), and hydrogen deuterium exchange MS (HDX-MS).[2,19-21] CD is a technique that measures the differences in the way proteins (e.g., a biosimilar versus an originator reference product) absorb left-handed and right-handed circularly polarized light.[20] By evaluating such differences, details about the secondary and tertiary structure of a protein can be elucidated.[2] The use of ultraviolet (UV) light in the far region (or far UV-CD) provides information about α-helices and β-sheets.[2] The use of UV light in the near spectrum (or near UV-CD) helps elicit information concerning the tertiary structure of a biologic given the intrinsic fluorescence of aromatic

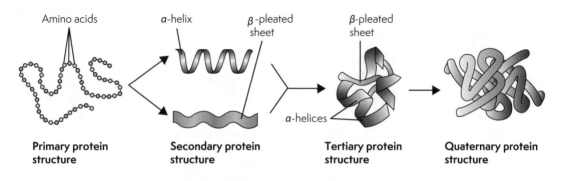

Amino acids   α-helix   β-pleated sheet   β-pleated sheet

α-helices

Primary protein structure   **Secondary protein structure**   **Tertiary protein structure**   **Quaternary protein structure**

FIGURE 4-3. LEVELS OF PROTEIN STRUCTURE.[40,41]

amino acids tryptophan, tyrosine, and phenylalanine.[2] Alternatively, secondary structures can be assessed through the application of infrared light in FTIR.[20] With this assay, the absorption of infrared light produces changes in the vibrational states of the biologic sample.[21] These vibrations provide a signature for the molecule that offers details concerning its secondary structure, allowing for comparison to a reference product.[20,21]

Another analysis is MS (HDX-MS).[19] Deuterium is a hydrogen isotope that contains one proton and one neutron, as compared to the most common form of hydrogen that has just one proton. In HDX-MS, a protein, such as an originator biologic or biosimilar, is exposed to deuterated water (D2O), which allows for an exchange of deuterium for hydrogen atoms.[19] This exchange is a function of the protein's structure as well as its dynamics. Where the exchange occurs, the heavier deuterium atom introduces additional mass that can be measured through MS to provide information regarding the structure of the protein and any changes in its confirmation.[19] Both originator biologics and biosimilars can be crystallized. Application of x-rays to these samples creates a diffraction pattern than can be compared to identify potential differences.[22] The way in which a protein behaves under stress also conveys information about its structure. In differential scanning calorimetry (DSC), heat is applied to a biologic. Any differences in the structure of the biologic would be reflected in its response to the application of heat.[12,18] In monoclonal antibodies and in other types of biologics, the presence of disulfide bonds is critical to ensure the appropriate structural conformation of the protein. Any variations could alter the biosimilars' performance. The use of Ellman's reagent, which binds to free thiol groups, enables the identification of disulfide bonds that failed to form, which could signal a change in the architecture of a proposed biosimilar.[32]

Post-translational Modifications

Among the most important characteristics involving biologic pharmaceuticals are the presence and activity of PTMs.[19] As their name implies, PTMs are chemical alterations to a protein that affect its structure and function. Common PTMs include acetylation, acylation, amidation, disulfide bond formation, glycosylation, phosphorylation, proteolytic processing, and sulfation.[40] Although all types of PTMs are significant in relation to any specific molecule, as a whole, glycosylation tends to be of greater concern given the frequency that this specific modification appears within licensed biopharmaceuticals.[42] Glycosylation includes galactosylation, fucosylation, high mannose derivatives, and sialylation and can affect a biologic's protein folding, targeting, trafficking, ligand recognition and binding, biological activity, stability, half-life, and immunogenicity.[19,42]

As in the case of assessing the amino acid sequence of a protein, both chromatography techniques and MS are essential tools to support assessment of PTMs and evaluation of any potential heterogeneity between biologic molecules.[2,12,20] Just as these tools can be used to create a peptide map of amino acids that connect to form a protein, they can create an oligosaccharide map that describes the glycosylation profile of a biologic.[2,12,20]

Other mechanisms used to assess PTMs include ion exchange chromatography (IEC) and isoelectric focusing (IEF).[12] In IEC, a buffer is used to modify the pH within a sample such that a protein possesses either a net positive charge (cationic) or a net negative charge (anionic).[34] The sample is passed over an exchange resin that is either anionic or cationic.[34] Therefore, the ionic profile of the molecule will determine the extent to which it interacts with the resin.[34] This profile can be compared between different samples to assess comparability.[34] IEF is a technique to separate samples based on their isoelectric point (pI), the pH at which the protein has no net charge.[25] A charge is applied across a pH gradient. The sample to be investigated migrates until it reaches its pI and no longer has a net charge. This tool enables the identification of minor changes in PTMs.[25]

Aggregation

A major concern in manufacturing of biologics is the potential for these products to form aggregates.[19] These unintended states of the monomeric form can be reversible or irreversible.[19] More importantly, they can result in many negative results including reducing the actual dosing concentration of a drug.[19] The greatest concern with aggregates is their unpredictable ability to cause immunological responses, which in some cases could be life-threatening.[19] Size exclusion chromatography (SEC) is a common method to assess and characterize protein aggregates due to its simplicity, low cost, ease of use, and high speed. SEC separates molecules based on their size by filtration through a gel.[19] The gel consists of spherical beads containing pores of a specific size distribution.[26] Small molecules are captured in the pores and as a result their continuing flow is interrupted.[26] However, larger molecules do not enter the pores, but are eluted.[26] Thus, molecules are eluted in the order of decreasing molecular weight.[26]

Another test, analytical ultracentrifugation (AUC) utilizes centrifugal acceleration applied to a sample to separate out components of different sizes.[27] Aggregates will migrate to a different extent than monomers of the biologic.[27] Other methods to assess aggregation include sodium dodecyl sulfate-polyacrylamide gel electrophoresis (SDS-PAGE) and capillary electrophoresis-sodium dodecyl sulfate (CE-SDS).[28,35] In SDS-PAGE, proteins are separated by mass because an ionic detergent, SDS, denatures and binds to proteins and renders them evenly negatively charged.[28] When a current is applied, all the SDS-bound proteins will move in a gel toward a positively charged electrode.[2] Lower mass proteins travel more quickly through the gel. This capability is particularly useful in evaluating aggregation as one of the primary differences between an aggregated product and the monomeric form would be the mass of the respective molecules.[28] CE-SDS is a similar and advanced technique.[35] Rather than utilizing a gel slab to separate molecules, this newer test utilizes gel in capillary columns.[35] CE-SDS is a more automated system that provides greater resolution and speed.[35]

The separation provided by electrophoresis can be combined with other technologies to enable identification of isolated proteins. One such technique is Western blotting.[29,36] After electrophoretic separation, proteins in a gel matrix can be bound to membranes where they are fixed and accessible for identification.[29,36] Western blotting combines the resolution of gel electrophoresis with the specificity of immunoassays.[36] A more gentle process, field flow fractionation (FFF), can be used to identify proteins of various sizes.[27] FFF is a single phase chromatography technique in which a suspension or solution is pumped through a long and narrow channel while at the same time a field is applied perpendicular to the flow of the liquid.[2] Particles of differing sizes flow at different rates and begin to separate. With FFF, there is no stationary phase thus limiting the potential for shearing or degradation of the sample.[27]

THE BENEFIT OF PREVIOUS EXPERIENCE

Obviously, there are many assays to evaluate the structure of biologic molecules and these tests are used in tandem, or orthogonally, to elucidate information concerning biosimilar molecules. It is important for us to understand the breadth of technologies. It is also critical to note that while these tests can find novel characteristics of biosimilar candidates, there are specific variations that have been identified as problematic during the development of originator reference products.[18,19]

The history of originator biologic drug development and comparability studies has created a wealth of information concerning biologic characteristics that can be particularly problematic.[18,19] Biosimilar developments must guard against numerous previously identified problems and have confirmatory evidence that specific signature issues do not exist in their proposed products. One example relates to small changes in the structure of a single amino acid and its ability to alter the immune tolerance of a biologic. Such is the case with the formation of iso-aspartic acid (isoAsp).[18,19] The development of this amino acid, either from the isomerization of aspartic acid or the deamidation of asparagine, has been shown to increase the immunogenic potential of proteins.[18,19] Careful scrutiny is required using technology such as MS.[18] Other amino acids that similarly draw attention include methionine, tryptophan, and histidine as these molecules are sensitive to oxidation, which can impact protein activity and stability.[17]

The higher order structure of a biologic is extremely influential to not only the efficacy of a product, but also the stability of the molecule and its capacity to remain viable under different storage conditions. Disulfide bonds are a critical component of the molecule infrastructure to ensure that protein folding occurs accurately.[2,32] Biosimilar manufacturers have the benefit of knowing which disulfide bonds are critical to preserving the biologic's functionality.[2,32]

Finally, variations in the presence and occurrence of PTMs, including glycosylation, phosphorylation, amidation, and sulfation, can alter the activity and safety of biologics.[42] For example, changes in the glycosylation of cetuximab have been associated with anaphylactic reactions.[19] Also, the presence of a specific sialic acid, N-glycolylneuraminic acid, also known as Neu5Gc or NGNA, has been associated with immunogenicity issues in monoclonal antibodies.[19] Any biosimilar application must account for potential issues identified in the development of the originator reference biologic.

LIGAND CONJUNCTION, WHAT'S YOUR FUNCTION?

The analytical tests that have been described thus far have primarily centered on the evaluation and description of the physical properties of biologic drugs, including the way amino acid sequences are ordered, how the protein folds, and any additional heterogeneity to the structure.[11] While all of these elements are extremely important, a biosimilar evaluation must also include an assessment of the protein's function.[12] As with the structural assessments, information concerning the binding and overall function of a proposed biosimilar are considered part of the totality of the evidence approach to approval.[13]

Similar to the techniques described above, many assays exist to evaluate the functional performance of a biosimilar.[2,11,12,16,18] To appreciate how these tests work, we must understand additional details regarding how biologic drugs exert their clinical effects. To put this into context, we will examine the structure activity relationships involving an important class of biologics, the monoclonal antibodies (mAbs), and the impact of glycosylation PTMs on their functioning.[43]

There are many types of biologics beyond mAbs. Nevertheless, the structural complexity of mAbs as well as the extent to which they are used in healthcare makes them excellent examples to describe the process of biosimilar functional characterization.[43] To understand the assays in question, we must remind ourselves of some basic elements of mAb construction. These biologics consist of two primary regions, the fragment antigen-binding (Fab) region and the fragment crystallizable (Fc) region.[43-45] As the name implies, the Fab region exerts its effects through antigen binding.[45] Alternatively, the Fc region interacts with cell surface receptors, called Fc receptors, and components of the complement system.[44] Depending on the mAb in question, these regions contribute to varying extents to the molecule's clinical efficacy.[43]

The mAbs are further differentiated by their chains, two heavy chains and two light chains.[45,46] As seen in **Figure 4-4**, each heavy chain consists of four domains, one variable and three constant.[45,46] Each light chain contains one constant and one variable region.[45,46] In addition, two disulfide bonds within the hinge region connect the heavy chains to each other, two disulfide bonds connect the heavy chains to the light chains, and 12 intrachain disulfide bonds further support the confirmation of the molecule.[45,46] Finally, important glycosylation related to mAb activity occurs within the second constant domain (CH2) of the Fc region.[45] The primary structure, higher order arrangement, associated PTMs, and any potential variation in the molecule must be identified and understood using the assays described previously.[45] **Figure 4-5** provides additional detail regarding the structural activity of a mAb.[44]

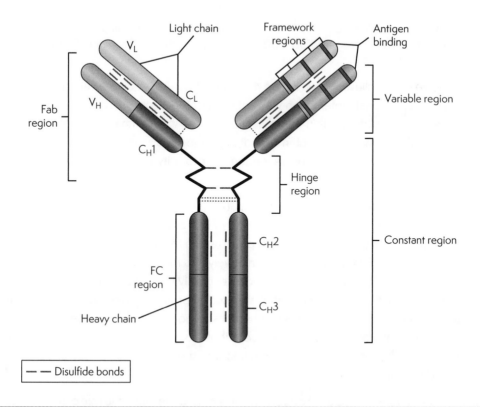

FIGURE 4-4. MONOCLONAL ANTIBODY STRUCTURE.[45,46]

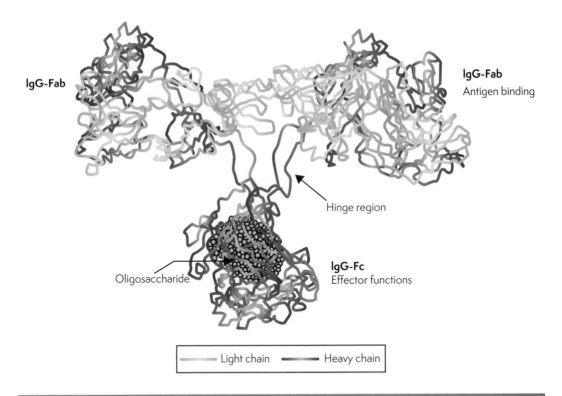

FIGURE 4-5. DETAILED REPRESENTATION OF A MONOCLONAL ANTIBODY.

Source: Reprinted from: Jefferis R. Recombinant antibody therapeutics: the impact of glycosylation on mechanisms of action. *Trends Pharmacol Sci.* 2009; 30:356-62. With permission from Elsevier.

As the more detailed illustration in Figure 4-5 reflects, a mAb requires a very specific conformation to ensure appropriate interaction with antigens or receptors.[44] In addition, the presence and influence of glycosylation within the Fc section of a mAb and the number of activities that are associated with binding in this region including phagocytosis, antibody-dependent cellular cytotoxicity (ADCC), and complement-dependent cytotoxicity (CDC) make evaluation of this area extremely important.[43]

We will use the example of the mAb rituximab to tie these concepts of Fab and Fc functioning together. In the graphical representation in **Figure 4-6**, the activities of both the Fab and Fc region on rituximab are shown.[44] It is the Fab region that binds the target CD20 receptor resulting in apoptosis of B lymphocytes.[44] Alternatively, it is the Fc region of the mAb that mediates ADCC and CDC.[44] It is within the Fc region, specifically the CH2 domain, where glycosylation (a PTM) can occur.[44] The side chains that are usually formed are described below in **Figure 4-7** where the normal core structure seen in humans is shown in bold.[44] However, other sugar residues, shown in light gray, are possible and contribute to the formation of hundreds of various combinations.[44] It is the variation in types and number of sugar moieties that can affect the functioning of a mAb, specifically the Fc region.[44]

Finally, to complete the circle of Fc interaction we must understand the role of the Fc receptor on effector cells like macrophages or natural killer (NK) cells. Within humans there are four types

CD20
Rituximab
(a)
Cytotoxic effector cell
(macrophage, NK)
(b)
FcγRIIIa
B lymphocyte
(c)
Complement Clq

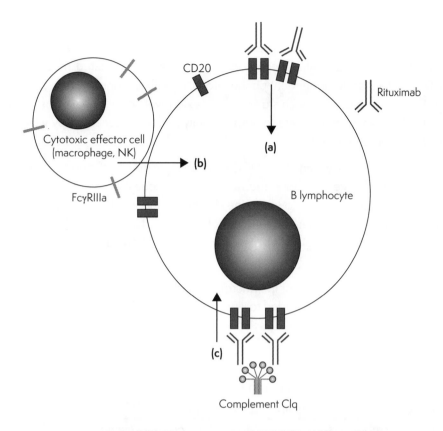

FIGURE 4-6. EFFECTS OF FAB AND FC BINDING ON MONOCLONAL ANTIBODY ACTIVITY (RITUXIMAB EXAMPLE).

Source: Reprinted from: Jefferis R. Recombinant antibody therapeutics: the impact of glycosylation on mechanisms of action. *Trends Pharmacol Sci.* 2009; 30:356-62. With permission from Elsevier.

Neu5Ac – Gal – GlcNAc – Man
Fuc
α(1–6) arm
GlcNAc – Man – GlcNAc – GlcNAc – Asn297
α(1–3) arm
Neu5Ac – Gal – GlcNAc – Man

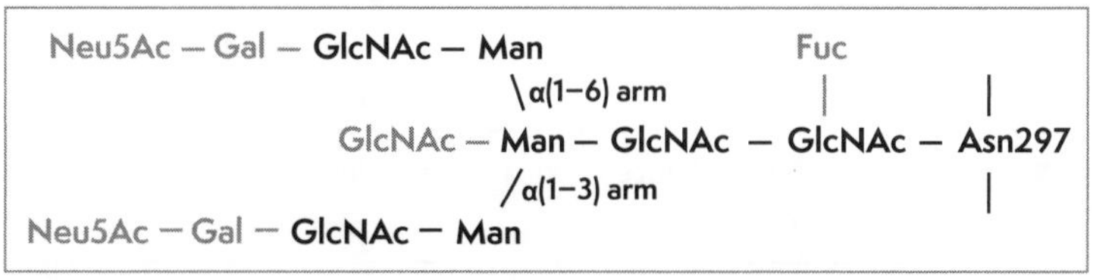

FIGURE 4-7. VARIATIONS IN GLYCOSYLATION OF FC REGION IN MONOCLONAL ANTIBODIES.

Source: Reprinted from: Jefferis R. Recombinant antibody therapeutics: the impact of glycosylation on mechanisms of action. *Trends Pharmacol Sci.* 2009; 30:356-62. With permission from Elsevier.

of Fc receptors of immune globulin G (IgG) molecules, FcγRI (also known as CD64), FcγRII (CD32 a, b, and c), FcγRIII (CD16 a,b, and c) and neonatal Fc receptor (FcRn).[47] FcγRI, FcγRIIa, FcγRIIc, and FcγRIIIa are activating receptors that induce cell-mediated responses including ADCC, CDC, and antibody-dependent phagocytosis. FcγRIIb is an inhibitory receptor. Of these receptors, FcγRIII has probably been studied more extensively given the role of FcγRIIIa in NK activity and ADCC, which both relate to autoimmunity and the mechanism by which oncology mAbs exert their therapeutic effect.[47]

One specific example involving the ADCC functioning of mAbs is the presence or absence of fucose.[47] As shown in Figure 4-7 above, fucose is a sugar residue that can attach to the N-acetyl-glucosamine (GlcNAc) subunit.[44] However, the absence of fucose alters Fc/Fc receptor binding such that ADCC activity increases on the order of 50 fold.[47] Therefore, a change in the glyco-sylation pattern within the Fc region can greatly alter the functioning of a mAb as referenced in **Table 4-2**.[47,48]

There are many PTMs that affect the pharmacokinetics and pharmacodynamics of biologic drugs. The above examples are intended to illustrate the extent to which minor changes can alter the behavior of recombinant proteins. As a result, rigorous testing of biologic activity is required when evaluating a biosimilar.[11,12,16,49-52]

TABLE 4-2. Impact of Glycosylation on the Pharmacokinetics and Pharmacodynamics of mAbs and Fc-Fusion Proteins[47,48]

Glycan	Efficacy/Safety/Immunogenicity	Clearance (PK/PD)
Mannose	■ Enhances FcγRIIIa binding/ADCC of mAb ■ Reduces C1q binding/CDC of mAb	■ Increases the clearance of mAb
Fucose	■ Interferes with binding to FcγRIIIa ■ Defucosylation enhances FcγRIIIa binding/ADCC activity	■ Unknown
Galactose	■ Enhances CDC of mAb	■ Exposed galactose may increase the clearance of mAb
GlcNAc	■ Bisecting GlcNAc enhance FcγRIIIa binding/ADCC	■ Increases the clearance of Fc-fusion proteins
Sialic acid NANA	■ Anti-inflammatory activity	■ Critical for reducing the clearance of Fc-fusion proteins
Sialic acid NGNA	■ Interferes with FcγRIIIa binding and reduces ADCC activity of mAb ■ May be immunogenic in humans	■ May affect drug clearance
Gal α1-3Galβ1-4GlcNAc-R	■ Immunogenic in humans and may induce anaphylaxis	■ Unknown

ADCC = antibody-dependent cellular cytotoxicity; CDC = complement dependent cellular cytotoxicity; NANA = N-acetylneuraminic acid; NGNA = N-glycolylneuraminic acid; GlcNAc = N-acetylglucosamine; Gal = galactose; Fc = fragment crystallizable; FcγR= IgG Fc receptor.

TABLE 4-3. Assays to Evaluate the Function of Biologics[11,12,16,49-51]		
Binding assays	■ Surface plasmon resonance (SPR) ■ ELISA ■ Biolayer interferometry ■ Cell-based assays	■ SPR—technique for measuring the binding of any pair of interacting molecules, including drugs and targets, antibodies and antigens (e.g., Fc receptor binding). Interactions are measured in real time enabling the determination of kinetic parameters. As binding occurs, the way in which light is reflected back to a detector changes allowing for characterization of the extent of interaction between the biologic and the receptor. ■ Biolayer interferometry—similar to SPR, but less affected by the refractive index of the sample being tested ■ ELISA—technique that evaluates the degree of antibody binding to an antigen usually through changes in color to denote the degree of interaction ■ Cell-based assays—cell lines developed to measure a biologic's activity based on receptor interaction
In vitro biological activity/mechanism of action	■ ELISA ■ Biolayer interferometry ■ Cell-based assays	■ Many of the same tests used in binding assays are deployed in the assessment of in vitro biological activity. Common attributes assessed for mAbs include evaluation of product's ability to mediate antibody-dependent cellular cytotoxicity, complement dependent cellular cytotoxicity, and apoptosis.

ELISA = enzyme-linked immunosorbent assay.

ASSESSING THE FAB VERSUS FC REGIONS IN PRACTICE

An increasing number of biosimilars are continuing to receive approval including versions of filgrastim, infliximab, adalimumab, and etanercept.[53] In each circumstance, FDA has concluded that the product met the standard of high similarity in conjunction with accompanying clinical trial data that confirmed the definition of biosimilarity.[54,55]

As seen in Figures 4-4 and 4-5, the function of the Fab and Fc regions can both be important to the functioning of the mAb.[44,45] The contribution of each of these regions to the activity of the molecule varies for every mAb. Within rheumatoid arthritis (RA)-related diseases, biologics such as infliximab and adalimumab exert their primary mechanism of action through the binding of both the soluble and transmembrane forms of the cytokine tumor necrosis factor tumor (necrosis factor-α [TNF-α]) through the Fab region as seen in **Table 4-4**.[54,55] The binding of TNF-α interrupts the inflammatory progression seen in RA, ankylosing spondylitis (AS), psoriatic arthritis (PsO), and plaque psoriasis (PsA).[54,55] This mechanism of action is likely also key in providing the treatment outcomes seen in Crohn's Disease (CD) and ulcerative colitis (UC).[54,55] In addition, the ability of infliximab and adalimumab to promote reverse signaling thus preventing apoptosis (cell death) and suppressing cytokine secretion is likely a critical function in CD and UC.[54,55] However, this effect is believed to be mediated through the Fab region of these mAbs.[54,55]

Conversely, the contribution of the Fc region to the treatment effect of infliximab and adalimumab is not as clear in the inflammatory bowel diseases.[54,55] Although it has been suggested the Fc region of these mAbs may be significant in regulating ADCC, CDC, and supporting mucosal healing, the evidence is not conclusive.[56] Nevertheless, given the need for thorough evaluation of all aspects of these molecules, both regions were analyzed as part of the application process for the biosimilar versions of infliximab and adalimumab.[54,55]

Analytical Characterization Results

In the analysis of infliximab-dyyb and adalimumab-atto, multiple tests demonstrated comparable binding and neutralization of TNF-α as compared to their originator reference counterparts suggesting that binding via the Fab regions of the molecules was in fact similar.[54,55] For adalimumab-atto, assessments of ADCC and CDC activity (plausible Fc-mediated mechanisms), were also comparable to the originator reference.[55] However, for infliximab-dyyb, an analytical assessment of ADCC using NK cells to measure activity appeared to reflect a slight difference.[54] In one test, 92% of the samples of infliximab-dyyb fell within the range of the originator compar-

TABLE 4-4. Mechanism of Action for Infliximab and Adalimumab in Licensed Inflammatory Conditions[55]

Mechanism of Action of Infliximab and Adalimumab	RA	AS	PsA	PsO	CD, Pediatric CD	UC, Pediatric UC
Mechanisms Involving the Fab (Antigen Binding) Region						
Binding and neutralization of s/tmTNF	Known	Known	Known	Known	Likely	Likely
Reverse (outside-to-inside) signaling via binding to tmTNF:	-	-	-	-	Likely	Likely
■ Apoptosis of lamina propria activated T cells	-	-	-	-	Likely	Likely
■ Suppression of cytokine secretion	-	-	-	-	Likely	Likely
Mechanisms Involving the Fc region						
■ Induction of CDC on tmTNF expressing target cells (via C1q binding)	-	-	-	-	Plausible	Plausible
■ Induction of ADCC on tmTNF-expressing target cells (via FcγRIIIa binding expressed on effector cells)	-	-	-	-	Plausible	Plausible
■ Induction of regulatory macrophages in mucosal healing	-	-	-	-	Plausible	Plausible

ADCC = antibody-dependent cellular cytotoxicity; AS = ankylosing spondylitis; CD = Crohn disease; CDC= complement dependent cellular cytotoxicity; PsA = plaque psoriasis; PsO = psoriatic arthritis; RA = rheumatoid arthritis; UC = ulcerative colitis.

ison.[54] As a result, FDA was required to assess whether or not this variation represented a meaningful difference.

In applying the totality of the evidence methodology, FDA concluded that this variation was not clinically significant.[54] First, a separate analysis of ADCC activity using peripheral blood mononuclear cells—a more diverse population than NK cells only and likely more representative of in vivo conditions—failed to show a difference between the biosimilar and the originator.[54] In addition, the other assessments of functional activity did not demonstrate a variation.[54] Finally, as articulated in Table 4-4, the activity of the Fc region of infliximab in inflammatory bowel diseases while plausible has not been definitively established.[54] FDA concluded that infliximab-dyyb met the standard of biosimilarity.[54] Given the comparability of structure and function between the originator and the biosimilar and the results of clinical trial data, FDA determined that infliximab-dyyb merited approval in not only the indications in which it was studied, RA and AS, but also indications such as CD and UC.[54] The European Medicines Agency made a similar determination when it approved the product in 2013.[45] Conversely, Health Canada initially declined to endorse this biosimilar for the inflammatory bowel disease indications in part based on these data.[45] Other mAbs for which biosimilars are under development, such as rituximab and trastuzumab, exert their clinical effects through the behavior of both the Fab and Fc regions.[43] Therefore, scrutiny of all physical and functional attributes of biosimilars will remain essential.

WHAT DOES ALL OF THIS MEAN FOR BIOSIMILARS?

After reviewing this discussion about analytical characterization, it is important to internalize two critical issues. First, the specificity and sensitivity of these techniques allows a thorough and rigorous scrutiny of biologic molecules at a level far beyond the extent to which a clinical trial can discern differences.[4] For example, these tests can differentiate between the influence of a hydrogen atom with one proton and a deuterium atom with a proton and a neutron.[19] The second consideration is the fact that the greater the quality of analytical characterization of the biosimilar, the smaller the clinical data package required to support approval.[3,4] In December 2016, FDA published the final version of its guidance document, "Clinical Pharmacology Data to Support a Demonstration of Biosimilarity to a Reference Product."[57] As shown in **Table 4-5**, FDA can reach one of four conclusions following characterization of a proposed biosimilar.[57] At one end of the spectrum, FDA can conclude that the molecule is so dissimilar, continuation of a 351(k) filing is not recommended. Conversely, the characterization phase could yield a finding of fingerprint-like analytical similarity, which would allow the biosimilar sponsor to pursue an increasingly targeted strategy for animal and/or clinical study design.[57] The size and scope of analytical characterization technologies coupled with confirmatory clinical trial data should enable prescribers and other clinicians to accept the stated safety and efficacy profile of licensed biosimilars.

TABLE 4-5. FDA Assessments of Similarity Following Analytical Characterization[57]

Assessment	Description of Findings
Insufficient analytical similarity	■ Further development via the 351(k) pathway is not recommended due to significant differences in the results of the analytical characterization process ■ Progression with 351(k) pathway would require changes to the manufacturing process for the proposed biosimilar
Analytical similarity with residual uncertainty	■ Additional information, analytical data, or other studies will be required to confirm that identified differences will fall into an acceptable range when the 351(k) application is submitted; e.g., subsequent pharmacokinetic and pharmacodynamic studies may demonstrate no clinically meaningful differences, thus mitigating concerns about residual uncertainties
Tentative analytical similarity	■ Results of analytical characterization allow for high confidence in the analytical similarity of the proposed biosimilar, and it can be appropriate for sponsor to conduct targeted and selective animal and/or clinical studies to address any residual uncertainty
Fingerprint-like analytical similarity	■ Results of characterization through a multi-parameter, extremely sensitive approach provides a very high level of confidence of analytical similarity; would be appropriate to conduct a more targeted and selective approach to subsequent animal and/or clinical studies

KEY POINTS

■ Analytical characterization forms the cornerstone of biosimilar development.

■ These tools and techniques allow for a rigorous evaluation of the structure and activity of biologic molecules and minimize the amount of clinical information needed to support biosimilar licensing.

■ Clinicians must understand and accept the sensitivity, specificity, and validity of these tools in ensuring biosimilars are clinically equivalent to branded biologics.

CONCLUSION

The biosimilar pathway does not exist in the absence of analytical characterization. The availability of numerous, detailed tools provides assurance that a comparable biologic product meets the same critical quality attributes as the originator and minimizes the level of clinical data to validate that similarity. Biosimilar evaluations have already demonstrated the validity of these tools and the capacity to lessen clinical trial requirements. Pharmacists must understand that a biosimilar approved in a highly regulated market such as the United States will have been rigorously scrutinized through a battery of such techniques. This appreciation will enable pharmacists to educate their fellow clinicians on the validity and utility of these tools.

REFERENCES

1. Singleton CA. MS in the analysis of biosimilars. *Bioanalysis.* 2014; 6:1627-37.

2. Kalman-Szekeres Z, Olajos M, Ganzler K. Analytical aspects of biosimilarity of protein drugs. *J Pharm Biomed Anal.* 2012; 69:185-95.

3. Weise M, Bielsky MC, De Smet K, et al. Biosimilars: what clinicians should know. *Blood* 2012; 120:5111-7.

4. McCamish M, Woollett G. The continuum of comparability extends to biosimilarity: how much is enough and what clinical data are necessary? *Clin Pharmacol Ther.* 2013; 93:315-7.

5. Chhina M. Biosimilar Biological Products. FDA basics webinar, August 19, 2013. https://www.fda.gov/downloads/AboutFDA/Transparency/Basics/UCM365448.pdf. (accessed Jul. 25, 2017).

6. McCamish M, Pakulski J, Sattler C, Woollett G. Toward interchangeable biologics. *Clin Pharmacol Ther.* 2015; 97:215-7.

7. Mulcahy AW, Predmore Z, Mattke S. The Cost Savings Potential of Biosimilar Drugs in the United States. RAND Corporation. www.rand.org/content/dam/rand/pubs/perspectives/PE100/PE127/RAND_PE127.pdf (accessed 3 Oct. 2017).

8. Express Scripts 2016 Drug Trend Report Executive Summary. February 2017. https://lab.express-scripts.com/lab/drug-trend-report (accessed 3 Oct. 2017).

9. Rathore AS. Quality by design (QbD)–based process development for purification of a biotherapeutic. *Trends Biotechnol.* 2016; 34:358-70.

10. Bui LA, Hurst S, Finch GL et al. Key considerations in the preclinical development of biosimilars. *Drug Discov Today.* 2015; 20 (suppl 1):3-15.

11. Al-Sabbagh A, Olech E, McClellan JE, Kirchhoff CF. Development of biosimilars. *Semin Arthritis Rheum.* 2016; 45(5 suppl):S11-8.

12. Tsuruta LR, Lopes dos Santos M, Moro AM. Biosimilars advancements: moving on to the future. *Biotechnol Prog.* 2015; 31:1139-49.

13. Quality considerations in demonstrating biosimilarity of a therapeutic protein product to a reference product. Guidance for industry. April 2015. www.fda.gov/downloads/drugs/guidancecompliance-regulatoryinformation/guidances/ucm291134.pdf (accessed 3 Oct. 2017).

14. Statistical approaches to evaluate analytical similarity. Guidance for industry, draft. September 2017. https://www.fda.gov/downloads/drugs/guidancecomplianceregulatoryinformation/guidances/ucm291134.pdf (accessed Oct. 3, 3017).

15. Shintani H. Development of test method for pharmaceutical and biopharmaceutical products. *Pharm Anal Acta.* 2013; 258:1-14.

16. Mestrovic T. What is mass spectrometry? www.news-medical.net/life-sciences/What-is-Mass-Spectrometry.aspx (accessed 3 Oct. 2017).

17. Federici M, Lubiniecki A, Manikwar P, Volkin DB. Analytical lessons learned from selected therapeutic protein drug comparability studies. *Biologicals* 2013; 41:131-47.

18. Alsenaidy MA, Jain NK, Kim JH et al. Protein comparability assessments and potential applicability of high throughput biophysical methods and data visualization tools to compare physical stability profiles. *Front Pharmacol.* 2014; 5:39.

19. Berkowitz SA, Engen JR, Mazzeo JR, Jones GB. Analytical tools for characterizing biopharmaceuticals and the implications for biosimilars. *Nat Rev Drug Discov.* 2012; 11:527-40.

20. Visser J, Feuerstein I, Stangler T et al. Physicochemical and functional comparability between the proposed biosimilar rituximab GP2013 and originator rituximab. *BioDrugs.* 2013; 27:495-507.

21. Fourier Transform Infrared Spectroscopy (FTIR). Materials Evaluation and Engineering, Inc. www.mee-inc.com/hamm/fourier-transform-infrared-spectroscopy-ftir/ (accessed 3 Oct. 2017).

22. Smyth MS, Martin JH. X-ray crystallography. *Mol Pathol.* 2000; 53:8-14.

23. Staub A, Guillarme D, Schappler J et al. Intact protein analysis in the biopharmaceutical field. *J Pharm Biomed Anal.* 2011; 55:810-22.

24. Ion exchange chromatography. Sigma-Aldrich. www.sigmaaldrich.com/life-science/proteomics/protein-chromatography/ion-exchange-chromatography.html (accessed 3 Oct. 2017).

25. Isoelectric focusing. ThermoFisher Scientific. www.thermofisher.com/us/en/home/life-science/protein-biology/protein-gel-electrophoresis/protein-gels/specialized-protein-gels/isoelectric-focusing.html (accessed 3 Oct. 2017).

26. Introduction to size exclusion chromatography. Bio-Rad. www.bio-rad.com/en-us/applications-technologies/introduction-size-exclusion-chromatography (accessed 3 Oct. 2017).

27. Liu J, Andya JD, Shire SJ. A critical review of analytical ultracentrifugation and field flow fractionation methods for measuring protein aggregation. *AAPS J.* 2006; 22:E580-9.

28. Overview of protein electrophoresis. ThermoFisher Scientific. www.thermofisher.com/us/en/home/life-science/protein-biology/protein-biology-learning-center/protein-biology-resource-library/pierce-protein-methods/overview-electrophoresis.html (accessed 3 Oct. 2017).

29. Kurien BT, Scofield RH. Western blotting: an introduction. *Methods Mol Biol.* 2015; 1312:17-30.

30. Introduction to capillary electrophoresis. Beckman Coulter. https://sciex.com/Documents/manuals/IntroductiontoCapillaryElectrophoresisVol-I.pdf (accessed 3 Oct. 2017).

31. Raynal B, Lenormand P, Baron B et al. Quality assessment and optimization of purified protein samples: why and how? *Microb Cell Fact.* 2014; 13:180.

32. Trivedi MV, Laurence JS, Siahaan TJ. The role of thiols and disulfides in protein chemical and physical stability. *Curr Protein Pept Sci.* 2009; 10:614-25.

33. Giri D. High performance liquid chromatrography (HPLC): principle, types, instrumentation and applications. http://laboratoryinfo.com/hplc/ (accessed 3 Oct. 2017).

34. Ion exchange chromatography. Bio-Rad. www.bio-rad.com/en-us/applications-technologies/liquid-chromatography-principles/ion-exchange-chromatography (accessed 3 Oct. 2017).

35. Den Engelsman J, Garidel P, Smulders R, et al. Strategies for the assessment of protein aggregates in pharmaceutical biotech product development. *Pharm Res.* 2011; 28:920-33.

36. Introduction to Western Blotting. Bio-Rad. www.bio-rad.com/en-us/applications-technologies/introduction-western-blotting (accessed 3 Oct. 2017).

37. Steen H, Mann M. The ABC's (and XYZ's) of peptide sequencing. *Nat Rev Mol Cell Biol.* 2004; 5:699-711.

38. Guevremont R, Kolakowski B. Using FAIMS to increase selectivity for LC-MS analyses. http://www.americanlaboratory.com/913-Technical-Articles/19191-Using-FAIMS-to-Increase-Selectivity-for-LC-MS-Analyses/ (accessed 3 Oct. 2017).

39. Beck A, Debaene F, Diemer H et al. Cutting-edge mass spectrometry characterization or originator, biosimilar, and biobetter antibodies. *J Mass Spectrom.* 2015; 50:285-97.

40. Protein structure. Particle Sciences, Drug Development Services. Technical Brief 2009, Volume 8. www.particlesciences.com/docs/technical_briefs/TB_8.pdf (accessed 3 Oct. 2017).

41. Biology LibreTexts. Proteins. https://bio.libretexts.org/TextMaps/Map%3A_Microbiology_(OpenStax)/07%3A_Microbial_Biochemistry/7.4%3A_Proteins (accessed 3 Oct. 2017).

42. Walsh G, Jefferis R. Post-translational modifications in the context of therapeutic proteins. *Nat Biotechnol.* 2006; 24:1241-52.

43. Jiang XR, Song A, Bergelson S et al. Advances in the assessment and control of the effector functions of therapeutic antibodies. *Nat Rev Drug Discov.* 2011; 10:101-11.

44. Jefferis R. Recombinant antibody therapeutics: the impact of glycosylation on mechanisms of action. *Trends Pharmacol Sci.* 2009; 30:356-62.

45. Scott BJ, Klein AB, Wang J. Biosimilar monoclonal antibodies: a Canadian regulatory perspective on the assessment of clinically relevant differences and indication extrapolation. *J Clin Pharmacol.* 2015; 55(suppl 3):S123-32.

46. Hansel TT, Kropshofer H, Singer T et al. The safety and side effects of monoclonal antibodies. *Nat Rev Drug Discov.* 2010; 9:325-38.

47. Liu L. Antibody glycosylation and its impact on the pharmacokinetics and pharmacodynamics of monoclonal antibodies and Fc-fusion proteins. *J Pharm Sci.* 2015; 104:1866-84.

48. Reusch D, Tejada ML. Fc glycans of therapeutic antibodies as critical quality attributes. *Glycobiology* 2015; 25:1325-34.

49. Hulse J, Cox C. SPR and flow cytometry for biosimilars. www.contractpharma.com/issues/2013-05/view_features/spr-flow-cytometry-for-biosimilars (accessed 3 Oct. 2017).

50. Perkel JM. Surface plasmon resonance (SPR) and other options for label-free detection. www.biocompare.com/Editorial-Articles/41803-Surface-Plasmon-Resonance-SPR-and-Other-Options-for-Label-free-Detection/ (accessed 3 Oct. 2017).

51. An introduction to ELISA. What is ELISA, procedures, types of ELISA, detection options and result. Bio-Rad. www.bio-rad-antibodies.com/an-introduction-to-elisa.html (accessed 3 Oct. 2017).

52. Lamerdin J, Daino-Laizure H, Charter NW, Saharia A. Acclerating biologic and biosimilar drug development: ready-to-use, cell-based assays for potency and lot-release testing. BioProcess International. www.bioprocessintl.com/upstream-processing/assays/accelerating-biologic-and-biosimilar-drug-development-ready-to-use-cell-based-assays-for-potency-and-lot-release-testing/ (accessed 3 Oct. 2017).

53. Drugs@FDA. FDA approved drug products. http://www.accessdata.fda.gov/scripts/cder/daf/ (accessed 3 Oct. 2017).

54. FDA briefing document. Arthritis Advisory Committee Meeting. February 09, 2016. BLA 125544. CT-P13, a proposed biosimilar to Remicade (infliximab), Celltrion. www.fda.gov/downloads/AdvisoryCommittees/CommitteesMeetingMaterials/Drugs/ArthritisAdvisoryCommittee/UCM484859.pdf (accessed 3 Oct. 2017).

55. FDA briefing document. Arthritis Advisory Committee Meeting. July 12, 2016. BLA 761024. ABP 501, a proposed biosimilar to Humira (adalimumab), Amgen. www.fda.gov/downloads/AdvisoryCommittees/CommitteesMeetingMaterials/Drugs/ArthritisAdvisoryCommittee/UCM510293.pdf (accessed 3 Oct. 2017).

56. Ben-Horin S, Vande Casteele N, Schreiber S, Lakatos PL. Biosimilars in inflammatory bowel disease: facts and fears of extrapolation. *Clin Gastroenterol Hepatol.* 2016; 14:1685-96.

57. Clinical pharmacology data to support a demonstration of biosimilarity to a reference product. Guidance for industry. December 2016. https://www.fda.gov/downloads/drugs/guidancecomplianceregulatoryinformation/guidances/ucm397017.pdf (accessed Oct. 3, 2017).

CHAPTER 5

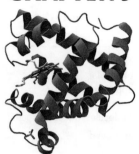

THE GLOBAL BIOSIMILARS EXPERIENCE

As the biosimilars market has continued to develop in the United States, pharmacists and other clinicians are likely cognizant that many of these products have been approved in other parts of the world. Other highly regulated markets in which biosimilars are currently licensed include Australia, Canada, Japan, South Korea, and most notably the European Union, which through the efforts of the European Medicines Agency (EMA), has entered its second decade of biosimilar development and use.[1-6] While none of these markets exactly resemble that of the United States, we can glean a substantial amount of information regarding the factors that influence the acceptance, prescribing, and use of biosimilars, and ideally avoid the previously identified barriers that could slow our adoption.[7] It is important to note that in these highly regulated markets where biosimilars are rigorously scrutinized prior to approval, these products have performed as expected with comparable safety and efficacy to their originator reference counterparts.[8,9]

AN OVERVIEW OF EUROPEAN EXPERIENCE

Highly-scrutinized, comparator versions of originator biologics (i.e., biosimilars) have been approved by many regulatory agencies across the globe.[1-6] The European market is the most mature both in terms of the duration of years biosimilars have been in existence as well as the number of products approved.[1] However, other markets have made significant contributions. For example, while the South Korean biosimilars market did not begin until 2012, the first biosimilar licensed was the Celltrion version of infliximab.[5] This product represented the first biosimilar monoclonal antibody approved in one of these highly regulated markets.[1-6] This biosimilar has since been licensed and marketed in both Europe and the United States (i.e., infliximab-dyyb).[1-6] The biosimilars approved in other nations are summarized in **Table 5-1**.[1-6]

Of all the global biosimilars markets, experience with these products is most substantial in Europe.[1] A legislative pathway for biosimilars in Europe was created in 2004, followed by an overarching regulatory guidance in 2005 leading to the first approved biosimilar, a version of somatropin, in 2006.[11,12] Europe has made the most progress in the development of biosimilars as they were the first to receive regulatory authority to approve such products and because significant patents that could have limited competition expired earlier as compared to markets such as the United States.[11] Since their initial introduction, multiple biosimilars have been approved across a range of categories from non-glycosylated agents, such as filgrastim and somatropin, through more complicated products such as fusion proteins and monoclonal antibodies.[1] With approximately a decade of experience, biosimilars have behaved as expected in terms of providing safe and effective alternatives to commonly used biologics and have helped to lower the overall cost of therapy and expand access to treatment.[9,13-15]

TABLE 5-1. Biosimilars Approved in Other Countries (Through July 2017)[1-6]

	EU	Australia	Canada	Japan	South Korea	U.S.
Year first biosimilar approved	2006	2010	2009	2009	2012	2015
Molecules approved	Adalimumab (1) Enoxaparin (2)* Epoetin (5) Etanercept (2) Filgrastim (7) Follitropin alfa (2)* Infliximab (3) Insulin glargine (2)* Insulin lispro (1)* Rituximab (6) Somatropin* Teriparatide (2)*	Epoetin (3) Etanercept (1) Filgrastim (3) Follitropin alfa (1)* Infliximab (2) Insulin glargine (1)* Somatropin (2)*	Etanercept (1) Filgrastim (1) Infliximab (2) Somatropin (1)*	Darbepoetin (1) Epoetin (1) Filgrastim (3) Infliximab (1) Insulin glargine (2)* Somatropin (1)*	Etanercept (2) Infliximab (2) Somatropin (1)* Rituximab (1) Trastuzumab (1)	Adalimumab (2) Bevacizumab (1) Etanercept (1) Filgrastim (1) Infliximab (2)
Total products approved	36	13	5	9	7	7

EU = European Union; U.S.= United States.

Note: Numbers in parentheses indiciate number of biosimilars of same molecule.

*Although approved as biologics in other nations, these products are presently approved in the United States as small molecule. Therefore, follow-on versions are not considered biosimilars.[10]

The track record of experience with certain European products has provided an additional measure of insight as biosimilars such as filgrastim-sndz (Zarxio; Sandoz), infliximab-dyyb (Inflectra; Celltion/Pfizer), and tbo-filgrastim (Granix; Teva), which is not considered a biosimilar in the United States, have received Food and Drug Administration (FDA) licensing.[1,6] For example, at the time of U.S. licensing of filgrastim-sdnz, over 7 million patient days of safety experience had been established globally for this product.[16] Similarly, as of July 2015 there were 24,000 patient years of experience worldwide with CT-P13, now known in the United States as infliximab-dyyb.[17] As the results of the studies that supported European approval of these products were already published in the clinical literature, U.S. pharmacists and clinicians had information concerning their clinical performance even prior to FDA approval decisions.[6] Therefore, it is possible that the approval of subsequent biosimilars could happen sooner in Europe and yield clinical information prior to an FDA advisory committee hearing or even final licensing. Still, we must remain aware that not all biosimilars will enter the European landscape before the U.S. market.[1,6] Furthermore, the U.S. biosimilar approval process can be trusted to approve biosimilar products of similar safety and efficacy, even without additional information from use in other countries.[11]

The introduction of biosimilars in Europe and other highly regulated markets has confirmed that these agents can and do provide a clinically similar outcome in terms of safety and efficacy as compared to their originator counterparts.[11,14,15,17] This global experience can also educate us on what is financially possible from biologic competition.[15]

Financial Performance

It is important to acknowledge that the healthcare financing and payment processes differ substantially between the United States and the rest of the world, including the EU.[18] In most other nations, the government is the primary entity that finances healthcare and the use of medications.[18] Conversely, while the government plays a role in the United States through entities such as Medicare and Medicaid, the private payer is more influential.[18] Even with these differences, it is encouraging to note that biosimilar availability in Europe has resulted in lower costs and greater access to treatment.[15] One example of the benefit of biosimilars is illustrated in the United Kingdom's experience with filgrastim.[15] Following the introduction of biosimilar competition, the health authorities in England revised their guidelines to reflect the improved cost effectiveness of filgrastim and moved the use of this product to first-line status for chemotherapy-induced neutropenia.[15] From January 2009 (shortly after the launch of biosimilar filgrastim) until January 2014, the overall use of all versions of short-acting filgrastim increased 104%.[15] By minimizing the expense of this product, therapy was made available to a larger population of patients. This example is further illustrated with the use of epoetin across the EU as a whole as well as for certain European nations. From the launch of biosimilar epoetin through 2014, the EU saw an average increased volume of treatment days of 16% while the price per treatment day decreased 27%.[15] For Romania, Bulgaria, and the Czech Republic, the increase in the volume of treatment days was 263% coupled with a decrease in price of treatment of 50%.[15] In nations such as Romania, Bulgaria, and the Czech Republic, biosimilars represent not just alternatives to competition, but primary treatment options where therapy was previously very limited or unavailable.[15] Even among the more economically capable nations, the degree of uptake and extent of price changes varies substantially. For example, Germany has witnessed price decreases of 55% for epoetin and 27% for filgrastim.[15] In contrast, the decreases in Italy have been 13% for epoetin and 4% for filgrastim.[15]

What Has Contributed to Greater Uptake in Certain European Countries?

No one factor has defined the success of biosimilars across all European nations.[19,20] In fact, various analyses have yielded differing results concerning the strategies that most correlate with increased biosimilar use.[19,20] However, one element that appears to support improved utilization is incentive programs such as prescription quotas for biosimilars.[19,20] Germany, Italy, Sweden, and Belgium have implemented quotas to encourage the use of biosimilars.[19,20] Other related programs to encourage physician use of biosimilars within these countries include ongoing monitoring of prescription patterns, financial incentives and/or penalties related to biosimilar use, and prescription prescribing guidelines.[20] In addition to forces encouraging prescribing of biosimilars, several strategies regarding contracting and reimbursement have also been leveraged to expand use.[20,21]

One of these approaches is known as reference pricing.[21] With this methodology, government health authorities establish a reference price that will be paid for a group of products that are deemed therapeutically equivalent.[21] Manufacturers may choose to sell their specific drug at a cost above or below the reference price.[21] However, patients are responsible for any costs above that threshold.[21] Another related strategy is that of tendering, or competitive bidding.[22] With this approach, hospitals conduct a competitive bid for a product.[22] Given the introduction of biosimilars, healthcare institutions and administrators now have agents that compete directly with branded products. Through this tendering process, Norway has recognized discounts of up to 89% with biosimilar filgrastim and 69% with biosimilar infliximab as a result of those products winning the tender.[23] The government acting as the primary payer for healthcare services facilitates both reference pricing and tendering. Again, given the pricing we have seen with biosimilar filgrastim and infliximab, this degree of savings should not be expected in the United States.[24,25] However, these examples demonstrate that competition enables lower pricing for high-cost biologics provided regulatory authorities, healthcare providers, and physicians are consistent in their adoption and acceptance of biosimilars.

Although there has been some consideration that existing familiarity and use of the generic model could translate into a comparable acceptance of the biosimilar market, a recent analysis does not validate that sentiment.[20] In this review of the biosimilar uptake across 10 nations in Europe, the extent of generic use was negatively correlated with the use of biosimilars.[20] While the true elements that drive biosimilar use remain somewhat uncertain and necessitate further evaluation,[20] the EMA has repeatedly articulated the importanace of one issue, which should serve as a very instructional point for the U.S. market, the commitment to continued prescriber and clinician education.[7,8]

CLINICIAN (AND PHYSICIAN) EDUCATION AND UNDERSTANDING

In spite of the early entry into the biosimilars era relative to other countries, the uptake of these medications has been more modest than initially anticipated or desired.[7,15] This limited extent of uptake was attributed to concerns either expressed directly by clinicians or through professional practice organizations about various aspects of the biosimilar concept.[7] Several of the concerns expressed related to the safety and efficacy of biosimilars in "extrapolated" indications, uses not directly studied in clinical trials. A summary of current position statements from several European professional practice organizations can be found in **Table 5-2**.[26-31]

To address these concerns, the EMA authored two extremely influential publications to advance the understanding of the biosimilar paradigm.[7,8] In both articles, the Working Party on Similar Biologic Medicinal Products of the EMA attempted to address these concerns through a detailed description of the scientific principles governing biosimilar development.[7,8] The first publication enumerated seven frequent vocalized concerns related to the quality, safety, and efficacy of biosimilars and provided specific answers articulating how the biosimilar approval process was structured to address and mitigate these issues.[7] A second article further addressed the challenge of extrapolation and why it is scientifically justified to license a biosimilar for use even if there are not clinical trial data for the product in a specific indication.[8] Both articles have proven very useful in dealing with the lack of familiarity of these principles and have

TABLE 5-2. Examples of Biosimilar Position Statements and Guidelines from European Professional Organizations[26-31]

Organization	Recommendation Type	Summary of Recommendations
World Marrow Donor Association	Position statement	■ Recommends that biosimilars not be used for (peripheral blood cell) mobilization in normal donors unless the donor is followed on a study looking at this question with both the recipient and the donor providing appropriate consent. ■ Only when comprehensive data to confirm long-term safety and efficacy is available should use of G-CSF biosimilars be considered routine.
European Crohn's and Colitis Organization	Position statement	■ Clinical studies of equivalence in the most sensitive indication can provide the basis for extrapolation; data for the use of biosimilar in IBD can be extrapolated from another sensitive indication. ■ A biosimilar registered in the EU can be considered as efficacious as the reference product. ■ "Switching from the originator to a biosimilar in patients with IBD is acceptable." More data are needed "regarding reverse switching, multiple switching, and cross-switching among biosimilar IBD patients." ■ Switching to a biosimilar from an originator should involve discussion between physicians, nurses, pharmacists, and patients.
British Society of Gastroenterology	Prescribing guidance	■ Infliximab should be prescribed by brand name (i.e., Remicade, Remsima, Inflectra) and not by the international non-proprietary name. ■ For patients starting on infliximab, any of the three products can be prescribed. ■ Sufficient evidence exists to switch a patient stable on Remicade to the biosimilar (Remsima or Inflectra) at the same dose and dose interval after discussion with individual patients. ■ Automatic substitution at the pharmacy level without consulting the prescriber is not appropriate.

(continued)

TABLE 5-2. (Continued)

Organization	Recommendation Type	Summary of Recommendations
Italian Group for Inflammatory Bowel Disease (IG-IBD)	Position statement	■ A biosimilar agent with proven efficacy and safety for one indication is not necessarily effective and safe for other indications. ■ It is highly recommended that, when the reference drug is used to treat IBD, evidence of the biosimilar's efficacy and safety in this specific setting be obtained prior to marketing. ■ An IBD patient being effectively controlled with an original biopharmaceutical should not be switched to a drug claimed to be that drug's biosimilar until preliminary data supporting such changes have been reported. The change must be approved by the specialist prescribing the original biologic and implemented after obtaining the patient's written informed consent. ■ The IG-IBD favors the use of biosimilar agents, provided that they meet appropriate quality standards and that their safety and efficacy have been specifically verified in IBD patients.
British Society of Rheumatology	Position statement	■ All biologics, originator and biosimilars, should be prescribed by their brand name. ■ Prescribing decisions should be made on the basis of clinical effectiveness and patient safety, not solely as a measure to save money. ■ Substitution of a biosimilar for a brand should only occur with the consent of the prescribing clinician. ■ Prescribing decisions should be made in partnership with physicians. ■ Recommends that all patients starting or switching to biosimilars should be registered with the British Society for Rheumatology Biologic Register or other appropriate UK register.
European League Against Rheumatism	Treatment guidelines	■ Biosimilar disease modifying antirheumatic drugs (DMARDS) that are EMA-approved or FDA-approved have similar efficacy and safety as their respective brands and should be preferred if they are indeed appreciably cheaper than the originator, other biologic DMARDs or targeted synthetic DMARDs. ■ A biosimilar DMARD of any reference biologic originator DMARD should not be used if the respective originator (or another biosimilar of the same molecule) previously failed to induce sufficient efficacy or vice versa.

been referenced in over 50 other articles relating to biosimilars.[32] The EMA has further invested in educational endeavors through materials such as its recently published, "Biosimilars in the EU, Information guide for healthcare professionals."[9] This commitment to clinician education combined with the increased availability of biosimilars appears to be increasing prescribers' level of comfort with these agents.

The European Crohn's Colitis Organization (ECCO) recently published the results of an updated survey, which was initially conducted in 2013.[33] The ECCO surveyed its members again in 2015 to assess changes in the level of knowledge and degree of comfort with biosimilars and identified several significant differences.[33] In 2013, 28.7% of participants responded they were "a little confident" and 32.3% "were not confident at all" in prescribing biosimilars.[33] In 2015, those numbers had decreased to 10.2% and 9.3%, respectively.[33] Perspectives regarding biosimilar interchangeability and extrapolation across indications had improved as well.[33] In response to these findings and given the overall improved knowledge concerning biosimilars, the ECCO has since revised its position statement for biosimilar use in inflammatory bowel disease.[27] Most notably, the revised position statement endorses the concept of extrapolation and removes the expressed requirement for safety and efficacy data to be established in each use for which a biosimilar is licensed.[27,34]

EXTRAPOLATION, NAMING, AND INTERCHANGEABILITY

In addition to the clinical and economic aspects of biosimilars, it is important to understand the global approach to other regulatory and practice considerations that are still being constructed within the United States. As seen in **Table 5-3**, the approaches across the elements are both similar and different.[35,36]

In general, most global markets have a similar approach to extrapolation.[35,36] If there is scientific justification, the regulatory bodies allow the use of clinical data in one indication to justify licensing of use of the biosimilar in other circumstances.[35] In spite of this commonality, regulatory bodies may reach different conclusions even for the same biosimilar as in the case of CT-P13, infliximab from Celltrion.[37] While EMA granted indication coverage across all uses of the originator, the approval in Canada initially excluded the inflammatory bowel diseases.[38] Conversely, the approach for biosimilar naming is variable. In some nations, differentiation of the biosimilar from the originator is required. In the EU, while the commercial name, appearance, and packaging should differ, Europe applies the same international nonproprietary name to the biosimilar as the originator.[35]

Interchangeability and Substitution

Unlike the United States, other highly regulated markets do not specifically differentiate their biosimilars in terms of being appropriate or inappropriate for interchange.[35] Nevertheless, the perspectives and experiences around the world and especially in Europe continue to fuel this discussion.[39] We must also understand that there are two distinct concepts when we discuss interchangeability. One is the regulatory consideration that it is equally safe to interchange or "switch" a patient back and forth between an originator and a biosimilar as it would be to maintain therapy with the originator all along.[40] The second aspect involves the discretion of a non-prescriber, usually a pharmacist, to substitute a biosimilar for the originator without the intervention of the physician.[40]

TABLE 5-3. Comparative Approaches to Biosimilar Regulation[35,36]

Element	EU	Australia	Canada	Japan	South Korea	U.S.
Extrapolation	Extrapolation to other diseases and settings for which reference products have EMA approval is on a case-by-case basis	The guidelines adopt the same standards of extrapolation as the EU	Clinical data could be extrapolated to other indications for which rationales are sufficiently persuasive	Extrapolation to other indications of the reference product might be possible	In some circumstances, a biosimilar product might receive extrapolated authorization for other indications of the reference product	Indication extrapolation is possible on a case-by-case basis
Naming and labeling	Commercial name, appearance, and packaging should differ and INN should be the same for related biosimilars	A biosimilar's Australian Biological Name must include the active ingredient of the reference product, and a biosimilar identifier. The biosimilar's trade name must be clearly distinguishable from the reference product. This system differs from the EMA and WHO	The labeling (product monograph) for an SEB should be developed in consistency with the principles, practices, and processes outlined in the Guidance for industry: product monograph (2004)	The nonproprietary name of a biosimilar in Japan includes a name for the generic combination and refers to the name of the reference product	Not addressed	Biologic nonproprietary names (originator and biosimilar) to be differentiated by the addition of a four-letter, devoid of meaning suffix

(continued)

TABLE 5-3. (Continued)

Element	EU	Australia	Canada	Japan	South Korea	U.S.
Substitution	Substitution is determined at the member-state level; this topic is not addressed in EMA guidance	No automatic substitution	No automatic substitution	Substitution should be avoided during the post-marketing surveillance period	Not addressed	Interchangeable—the applicant has to show that the biological product can be expected to produce the same clinical result as the reference product in any patient. Biosimilars that are deemed interchangeable could be substituted for reference products without physicians' orders

EMA = European Medicines Agency; EU = European Union; INN = international nonproprietary names; SEB = subsequent entry biologics; U.S.= United States; WHO = World Health Organization.

Source: Reprinted with permission from Bennett CL, Chen B, Hermanson T, et al. Regulatory and clinical considerations for biosimilar oncology drugs. Lancet Oncol. 2014;15:e594-605.

Most regulatory bodies do not make a determination of when substitution should or should not happen.[35] The EMA specifically leaves the consideration of substitution to the discretion of member states, and most states have thus far declined to support such interchange.[35] In fact, 12 countries across the EU have introduced rules to prevent automatic substitution of biosimilars for the originator biologics.[35] However, France has recently taken the step to allow a restricted level of pharmacy-level substitution by a pharmacist when the physician has not prohibited such an interchange.[41]

Much conversation has taken place regarding the extent to which approved biosimilars can be interchanged or switched for the originator.[39] Based upon the review of available data in pre-approval clinical trials, published open label results, and registry information, licensed biosimilars from highly regulated markets appear to provide the same safety and efficacy results when switched for the originator reference product to which they are compared.[39,42] In a recent letter, representatives from several national regulatory agencies in Europe stated that based upon experience with currently marketed biosimilars and information in the literature, "switching patients from the originator to a biosimilar medicine or vice versa can be considered safe."[39]

DEVELOPING MARKETS AND SAFETY ISSUES

Products characterized as biosimilars have also been marketed and continue to be developed in the emerging markets segment.[43] Even though some of these products have performed as expected, there have also been reports of adverse events, such as pure red cell aplasia with versions of epoetin.[43] It must be recognized that these inferior products were not subjected to the rigorous standards of the EU or the United States.[44] As a result, these products do not meet the definition of biosimilars.[44] Although these products may meet a market need in countries where access to treatment is limited, we should not confuse these products or their adverse event profiles with the biosimilars that the FDA has approved or will ultimately approve.

KEY POINTS

- Biosimilars have been used safely and effectively in many markets, most notably in Europe. While still under development, the introduction of competing products has allowed for some cost savings and by extension, increased access to care.

- The biosimilar model in other markets continues to mature and different governments continue to implement multiple strategies to increase adoption.

- Clinician, particularly physician, education is critically important to sustaining acceptance and use of biosimilars.

CONCLUSION

The track record for biosimilars approved in the EU and other highly regulated markets validates the fact that such products can be used safely and effectively to lower costs and increase access. Such data should serve as an additional level of comfort for biosimilar acceptance. However, as global markets vary from the United States, it is important to apply lessons learned abroad within the context of our healthcare infrastructure. For example, the absence of a single payer system in the United States will likely limit the extent of cost savings as compared to what has been seen in some European countries. Still, many other aspects of the European experience are very useful in framing our ability to expand the acceptance of biosimilars in this country, particularly the essential need to ensure prescriber and clinician understanding and acceptance that govern the basic use of these medications.

REFERENCES

1. European Public Assessment Reports. Authorised biosimilars. www.ema.europa.eu/ema/index.jsp?curl=pages/medicines/landing/epar_search.jsp&mid=WC0b01ac058001d124&searchTab=-searchByAuthType&keyword=Enter%20keywords&searchType=name&alreadyLoaded=true&status=Authorised&jsenabled=false&searchGenericType=biosimilars&orderBy=name&pageNo=1 (accessed 3 Oct. 2017).

2. Biosimilars approved in Australia. www.gabionline.net/Biosimilars/General/Biosimilars-approved-in-Australia. (accessed 3 Oct. 2017).

3. Subsequent entry biologics approved in Canada. www.gabionline.net/Biosimilars/General/Subsequent-entry-biologics-approved-in-Canada (accessed 3 Oct. 2017).

4. Biosimilars approved in Japan. www.gabionline.net/Biosimilars/General/Biosimilars-approved-in-Japan (accessed 3 Oct. 2017).

5. Biosimilars approved in South Korea. www.gabionline.net/Biosimilars/General/Biosimilars-approved-in-South-Korea (accessed 3 Oct. 2017).

6. Drugs@FDA: FDA Approved Drug Products. www.accessdata.fda.gov/scripts/cder/daf/index.cfm (accessed 3 Oct. 2017).

7. Weise M, Bielsky MC, De Smet K et. al. Biosimilars: what clinicians should know. *Blood.* 2012; 120:5111-7.

8. Weise M, Kurki P, Wolff-Holz E et al. Biosimilars: the science of extrapolation. *Blood.* 2014; 124:3191-6.

9. EMA. Biosimilars in the EU. Information guide for healthcare professionals. http://www.ema.europa.eu/docs/en_GB/document_library/Leaflet/2017/05/WC500226648.pdf (accessed 3 Oct. 2017).

10. Food and Drug Administration. Guidance for industry, draft guidance. Implementation of the "Deemed to be a License" provision of the Biologics Price Competition and Innovation Act of 2009. www.fda.gov/downloads/drugs/guidancecomplianceregulatoryinformation/guidances/ucm490264.pdf (accessed 3 Oct. 2017).

11. McCamish M, Woollett G. Worldwide experience with biosimilar development. *MAbs* 2011; 3:209-17.

12. Goel N, Chance K. Biosimilars in rheumatology: understanding the rigor of their development. *Rheumatology (Oxford).* 2017; 56:187-97.

13. Kurki P, Ekman N. Biosimilar regulation in the EU. *Expert Rev Clin Pharmacol.* 2015; 8:649-59.

14. Schulz M, Bonig H. Update on biosimilars of granulocyte colony-stimulating factor—when no news is good news. *Curr Opin Hematol.* 2015; 23:61-6.

15. Delivering on the Potential of Biosimilar Medicines: The Role of Functioning Competitive Markets. IMS Health, March 2016. www.imshealth.com/files/web/IMSH%20Institute/Healthcare%20Briefs/Documents/IMS_Institute_Biosimilar_Brief_March_2016.pdf (accessed 3 Oct. 2017).

16. Novartis press release: FDA approves first biosimilar Zarxio (filgrastim-sndz) from Sandoz. www.biospace.com/News/novartis-ag-release-fda-approves-first-biosimilar/367742 (accessed 3 Oct. 2017).

17. Braun J, Kudrin A. Switching to biosimilar infliximab (CT-P13): Evidence of clinical safety, effectiveness and impact on public health. *Biologicals* 2016; 44:257-66.

18. Whalen J. Why the U.S. pays more than other countries for drugs. Norway and other state-run health systems drive hard bargains, and are willing to say no to costly therapy. www.wsj.com/articles/why-the-u-s-pays-more-than-other-countries-for-drugs-1448939481 (accessed 3 Oct. 2017).

19. Grabowski H, Guha R, Salgado M. Biosimilar competition: lessons from Europe. *Nat Rev Drug Discov.* 2014; 13:99-100. Supplementary information.

20. Remuzat C, Dorey J, Cristeau O et al. Key drivers for market penetration of biosimilars in Europe. *J Mark Access Health Policy.* 2017; 5:1-15.

21. Lee JL, Fischer MA, Shrank WH et al. A systematic review of reference pricing: implications for US prescription drug spending. *Am J Manag Care.* 2012; 18:e429-37.

22. Rompas S, Goss T, Amanuel S, et al. Demonstrating value for biosimilars: a conceptual framework. *Am Health Drug Benefits.* 2015; 8:129-39.

23. Asbjorn M. Norway, biosimilars in different funding systems. What works? www.gabi-journal.net/norway-biosimilars-in-different-funding-systems-what-works.html (accessed 3 Oct. 2017).

24. Johnson SR. One year after Zarxio approval, future of biosimilars remains unclear. www.modern-healthcare.com/article/20160323/NEWS/160319919 (accessed 3 Oct. 2017).

25. Pfizer announces the U.S. availability of biosimilar INFLECTRA (infliximab-dyyb). Press release. www.pfizer.com/news/press-release/press-release-detail/pfizer_announces_the_u_s_availability_of_biosimilar_inflectra_infliximab_dyyb (accessed 3 Oct. 2017).

26. Shaw BE, Confer DL, Hwang WY et al. Concerns about the use of biosimilar granulocyte colony-stimulating factors for the mobilization of stem cells in normal donors: position of the World Marrow Donor Association. *Haematologica* 2011; 96:942-7.

27. ECCO position statement on the use of biosimilars for inflammatory bowel disease-an update. *J Crohns Colitis.* 2017; 11:26-34.

28. BSG Guidance on the Use of Biosimilar Infliximab CT-P13 in IBD. www.bsg.org.uk/clinical/news/bsg-guidance-on-the-use-of-biosimilar-infliximab-ct-p13-in-ibd.html (accessed 3 Oct. 2017).

29. Annese V, Vecchi M, Italian Group for the Study of IBD (IG-IBD). Use of biosimilars in inflammatory bowel disease: Statements of the Italian Group for Inflammatory Bowel Disease. *Dig Liver Dis.* 2014;46:963-8.

30. The British Society of Rheumatology Biosimilars Position Statement, January 2017 revision. http://80.87.12.43/resources/bsr_biologics_registers/biosimilars.aspx?print=true#l1 (accessed 3 Oct. 2017).

31. Smolen JS, Landewe R, Bijlsma J et al. EULAR recommendations for the management of rheumatoid arthritis with synthetic biological disease-modifying antirheumatic drugs: 2016 update. *Ann Rheum Dis.* 2017; 76:960-77.

32. US National Library of Medicine. PubMed/Medline search. www.nlm.nih.gov/ (accessed 3 Oct. 2017).

33. Danese S, Fiorino G, Michetti P. Changes in biosimilar knowledge among European Crohn's Colitis Organization [ECCO] members: an updated survey. *J Crohns Colitis* 2016; 10:1362-5.

34. Danese S, Gomollon F, Governing Board and Operational Board of ECCO. ECCO position statement: the use of biosimilar medicines in the treatment of inflammatory bowel disease (IBD). *J Crohns Colitis.* 2013; 7:586-9.

35. Bennett CL, Chen B, Hermanson T et al. Regulatory and clinical considerations for biosimilar oncology drugs. *Lancet Oncol.* 2014; 15:e594-605.

36. Food and Drug Administration. Guidance for industry. Nonproprietary naming of biological products, January 2017. http://www.fda.gov/downloads/drugs/guidances/ucm459987.pdf (accessed 3 Oct. 2017).

37. Scott BJ, Klein AV, Wang J. Biosimilar monoclonal antibodies: A Canadian regulatory perspective on the assessment of clinically relevant differences and indication extrapolation. *J Clin Pharmacol*. 2015; 55(suppl 3):S123-32.

38. Ben-Horin S, Vande Casteele N, Schreiber S, Lakatos PL. Biosimilars in inflammatory bowel disease: facts and fears of extrapolation. *Clin Gastroenterol Hepatol*. 2016; 14:1685-96.

39. Kurki P, van Aerts L, Wolff-Holz E et al. Interchangeability of biosimilars: a European perspective. *BioDrugs*. 2017; 31:83-91.

40. Food and Drug Administration. Guidance for industry. Considerations in demonstrating interchangeability with a reference product, draft guidance, January 2017. https://www.fda.gov/downloads/Drugs/GuidanceComplianceRegulatoryInformation/Guidances/UCM537135.pdf (accessed 3 Oct. 2017).

41. Thimmaraju PK, Rakshambikai R, Farista R, Juluru K. Legislations on biosimilar interchangeability in the US and EU—developments far from visibility. www.gabionline.net/Sponsored-Articles/Legislations-on-biosimilar-interchangeability-in-the-US-and-EU-developments-far-from-visibility (accessed 3 Oct. 2017).

42. Moots R, Azevedo V, Coindreau JL et al. Switching between reference biologics and biosimilars for the treatment of rheumatology, gastroenterology, and dermatology inflammatory conditions: considerations for the clinician. *Curr Rheumatol Rep*. 2017;19:37.

43. Praditpornsilpa K, Tiranathanagul K, Kupatawintu P et al. Biosimilar recombinant human erythropoietin induces the production of neutralizing antibodies. *Kidney Int*. 2011;80:88-92.

44. Weise M, Bielsky MC, De Smet K et al. Biosimilars—why terminology matters. *Nat Biotechnol*. 2011;29:690-3.

CHAPTER 6

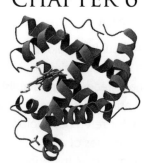

THE AMERICAN BIOSIMILAR EXPERIENCE: RED, WHITE, AND POSSIBLY INTERCHANGEABLE

The U.S. biosimilar era officially began on March 23, 2010 with the enactment of the Biologics Price Competition and Innovation (BPCI) Act, the statute that granted the Food and Drug Administration (FDA) authority to approve highly similar versions of previously licensed biologics.[1] The progress toward this step was neither easy nor quickly achieved, but instead necessitated over a decade of negotiation to translate the initial concept of competing biologics into a regulatory reality.[2] As is the case with any product of sustained legislative deliberation and compromise, the resulting regulatory authority has required additional time to allow for interpretation, sometimes by the courts, and continued implementation. Although several years have passed since initial enactment, various elements of the biosimilar pathway remain tentative or undefined. Still, many components have received greater clarity from FDA through both published guidance documents as well as a number of approval actions that continue to accrue and accelerate. This chapter describes the essential aspects of the approval mechanism for biosimilars, both final and provisional, and how the implementation of these requirements affects clinical practice.

AN OVERVIEW OF THE BPCI ACT

The BPCI Act established the overarching authority of FDA to approve biosimilars.[1] It further empowered the agency to clarify the details of the approval process via the publication of guidance documents and additional rule making actions.[1] Although many aspects concern the global approval process, two issues the BPCI Act explicitly defines for the U.S. market are the term *biosimilar* and the concept of *biosimilarity*.

According to the BPCI Act, these terms signify:

- "that the biological product is highly similar to the reference product notwithstanding minor differences in clinically inactive components"[1] and

- "there are no clinically meaningful differences between the biological product and the reference product in terms of safety, purity, and potency of the product"[1]

This definition articulates the aspirational goal of the BPCI Act that this regulatory pathway enables the review, validation, and approval of highly similar biologics that while not identical generic products (for the reasons described in Chapter 3), can be expected to result in the same clinical outcome (safety and efficacy) as a previously licensed branded biologic drug.[1]

A Novel Approach to Approving Something That Already Exists

Although the biosimilar approval process is new, its intended output is not. The end result of a successful biosimilar development program is a product whose clinical performance profile has already been established by an originator reference product.[1] The approval opportunity for biosimilars is limited to the authorization of highly similar versions of previously approved originator reference biologics and is not intended to support the licensing of novel products or novel uses of an existing product.[1] Biosimilars must utilize the same mechanism or mechanisms of action as the originator biologic, to the extent that this information is known.[1] A biosimilar can be approved only for "the condition or conditions of use prescribed, recommended, or suggested in the labeling" of the originator reference product.[1] The route of administration, the dosage form, and the strength of the biosimilar must be the same as that of the originator biologic.[1] Finally, the facility in which the biosimilar is manufactured, processed, packed, or held must support the safety, purity, and potency of the product.[1]

As described in Chapter 4 of this text, analytical studies are the foundational component of a biosimilars application and enable the approval of such products in a manner that is more efficient, yet still preserves safety and efficacy. These requirements are described in the text of the BPCI Act along with the animal studies (including the assessment of toxicity) and a clinical study or studies (including the assessment of immunogenicity and pharmacokinetics or pharmacodynamics) that also contribute to a biosimilar application.[1]

BPCI ACT HIGHLIGHTS

In addition to these requirements and limitations of a biosimilar application, the BPCI Act defines several other critical aspects of the approval process as described in **Table 6-1**.

Among these elements, the BPCI Act establishes the exclusivity period for originator biologics, where no such threshold previously existed. For example, FDA may not accept an application for a biosimilar until four years after the first approval of the originator. Furthermore, FDA cannot approve a biosimilar until 12 years after initial licensing of the originator. These timeframes have limited relevance for products currently nearing approval since their originator counterparts have already enjoyed more than 12 years of exclusivity given their existence prior to the statute's implementation. Still, for biologics approved since March 2010, the period of exclusivity has now been established. Biologic manufacturing is highly proprietary, creating substantial patent infringement opportunities. As such, the BPCI Act defines an approach to navigate these legal hurdles, although this mechanism itself continues to drive litigation that will be detailed further in Chapter 9. In keeping with the requirements of comparable safety, purity, and potency, biosimilars are subject to the same Risk Evaluation Mitigation Strategies as their branded counterparts. Finally, the BPCI Act includes some general parameters for defining biologic interchangeability, a topic that will be discussed in more detail later in this chapter.[1]

DEFINING THE SPACE BETWEEN GENERIC SMALL MOLECULES AND COMPARABLE BIOLOGICS

Another way to improve our understanding of the biosimilar approval pathway is to compare it with the other mechanisms by which medications are approved. The biosimilar pathway, also

TABLE 6-1. Additional Aspects of BPCI Act[1-4]

Element	Comments
Timing of application filing and originator exclusivity	■ FDA may not accept a biosimilar application until 4 years after the initial approval of the originator reference biologic ■ FDA may not approve a biosimilar until 12 years after the initial approval of the originator reference biologic
Patent litigation	■ The BPCI Act enumerates a detailed process often described as the patent dance to litigate potential infringements of originator patents. This process is itself the subject of litigation. ■ See Chapter 9 for more information on biosimilar litigation issues.
Transition of biologics previously licensed as drugs	■ Certain recombinant biologic products have previously been licensed through new drug applications rather than biologics license applications ■ 10 years following enactment of the BPCI Act (March 23, 2020), these products (e.g., insulin, somatropin) will now be considered biologics

Interchangeability	■ FDA may designate certain biosimilars as interchangeable, meaning that,
	
	  ● The product "can be expected to produce the same clinical result as the reference product in any given patient," and "for a biological product that is administered more than once to an individual, the risk in terms of safety or diminished efficacy of alternating or switching between use of the biological product and the reference product is not greater than the risk of using the reference product without such alternation or switch"
	
	  ● The interchangeable biologic may be substituted for the originator reference product without the intervention of the prescriber
	
	■ The BPCI Act also defines certain additional exclusivity for the first interchangeable biosimilar for an originator reference product.

Risk evaluation mitigation strategies (REMS)	■ Biosimilars are subject to REMS requirements just as their originator counterparts.

known as a 351(k) biologics license application (BLA), bears a resemblance to several other medication approval processes as listed in **Table 6-2**.[5]

Novel reference products are approved via the new drug application (NDA) or 505(b)1 pathway if a small molecule drug, or the 351(a) BLA pathway if a biologic medication.[2,5] Generic or other follow-on versions of originator small molecules may be approved via an abbreviated new drug application (ANDA), also known as the 505(j) process, or the 505(b)2 version of the NDA.[2,5] Finally, when an originator biologic undergoes a manufacturing change, validation that the medication's clinical performance remains unaltered by the modification is determined through the International Conference on Harmonization (ICH) Q5E standard.[6] The biosimilar 351(k) version of a BLA bears a resemblance to each of these last three mechanisms.

Similar to an ANDA-approved generic medication, a biosimilar is intended to serve as a competing version of a previously approved originator reference medication. Similar to the "A" therapeutic equivalency rating for generic medications, it is technically possible for FDA to desig-

TABLE 6-2. Approval Processes for Drug and Biologics[1,2,5]

Product Type (Governing Statute)	Application Type	Application Pathway	Clinical Studies Requirement	Resulting Approved Product
Drug (Food, Drug, and Cosmetic Act)	New Drug Application (NDA)	505(b)1	Yes, full evaluation of safety and efficacy	■ Small molecule, new molecular entity
		505(b)2	Yes, however, studies do not have to be done by the application sponsor	■ Hybrid approval pathway between 505(b)1 NDA and 505(j) ANDA ■ Allows for approval of new dosage form, strength, route of administration, or substitution of an active ingredient in a combination product ■ Can possibly receive an "A" therapeutic equivalency rating, but not always granted ■ Pathway has been used for approval of follow-on versions of recombinant biologics previously approved under NDA such as somatropin, insulin glargine, glucagon; such products are not currently considered biosimilars
	Abbreviated New Drug Application (ANDA)	505(j)	No, but must demonstrate bioequivalence	■ Generic medication ■ Exact copy of originator reference, small molecule drug ■ Usually granted an "A" therapeutic equivalency rating indicating the product is substitutable with the originator, branded drug
Biologic (Public Health Services Act)	Biologics License Application (BLA)	351(a)	Yes, full evaluation of purity, safety and potency	■ Novel, biologic molecular entity
		351(k)	Yes, but abbreviated process	■ Highly similar biologic to originator reference product ■ Potential for biosimilar to be designated as interchangeable, but requirements not yet defined

(continued)

TABLE 6-2. (Continued)

Product Type (Governing Statute)	Application Type	Application Pathway	Clinical Studies Requirement	Resulting Approved Product
Comparable biologic (International Conference on Harmonization Q5E Standard)	Comparability study		Clinical data may be required, but analytical characterization usually enough to validate comparability	■ Validates that originator, reference biologic is comparable to pre-change version following manufacturing change[6] ■ Product is treated as interchangeable, since there is no identification in the United States when biologic goes through manufacturing change and associated comparability determination[6]

nate a biosimilar as interchangeable.[1] The biosimilar pathway also bears similarities to the 505(b)2 approval mechanism given that this application requires submission of clinical data.[5] However, a 505(b)2 applicant can rely on the branded company's generated information whereas the biosimilar must conduct its own studies.[1,5] While products approved via a 505b(2) application may receive an "A" therapeutic equivalency rating, that is not always the case. Examples of products lacking the "A" rating include recombinant biologics whose originator reference products were initially approved as drugs such as somatropin and the various insulin presentations including aspart, lispro, glargine, and detemir.[6] Although these products are follow-on versions of previously approved biologics, they are currently not considered biosimilars. According to the BPCI Act, 10 years after enactment or March 23, 2020, such products will transition from regulation as drugs to biologics.[1]

Finally, the biosimilar pathway displays a commonality with the ICH Q5E standard used to determine comparability of originator reference biologics following manufacturing changes (described in more detail in Chapter 3).[6] Just as a branded company must show that its pre-change and post-change version of an originator molecule is comparable, a biosimilar must show that a different set of production steps can produce a highly similar molecule.[5,6] Given the originator's level of knowledge about the production process, both pre- and post-change, many comparability determinations can be based on analytical data alone.[5,6] Biosimilar applicants must always include some level of clinical data.[1] Still, analytical characterization is a shared, essential element of both comparability and biosimilarity.[1,6]

As a result, while the specific biosimilar pathway is new, many related principles of similarity, substitutability, and clinical data requirements have existed in the other mechanisms used to approve medications in the United States. Ideally, our level of familiarity and confidence in these existing approval mechanisms will translate into increasing comfort with the biosimilar regulatory process.

FILLING IN THE DETAILS—THE BIOSIMILAR GUIDANCES

One of the less controversial aspects of the BPCI Act was the inclusion of FDA's authority to publish guidance documents regarding the biosimilar approval pathway.[1] As of October 2017, FDA has published 12 guidances detailing numerous aspects regarding biosimilar approval. **Table 6-3** lists those guidances along with a summary of FDA's current thinking on various elements of the biosimilar process.

The number of guidances published further illustrates the challenge and complexity of bringing a new approval process into existence. FDA has had to address everything from its overall approach to biosimilar approval to details about the attributes associated with biosimilars (i.e., naming).[7,14] FDA encourages a stepwise approach—at each stage of development, the sponsor assesses what residual uncertainty regarding biosimilarity remains and what additional studies are required to address that uncertainty.[7] A companion concept furthered by FDA in the biosimilar approval process is the use of the totality of the evidence approach.[7] This principle means that rather than considering information from individual steps in isolation, FDA will evaluate the totality of evidence from analytical characterization, nonclinical evaluation, pharmacokinetic and pharmacodynamic studies, clinical immunogenicity data, and all comparative study information in determining the biosimilarity status of a proposed product.[7]

The guidances for scientific and quality considerations have played the most substantial role as they describe the approach to approval for clinical evaluation and analytical characterization, respectively.[7,8] The clinical pharmacology guidance is also very influential in helping describe how FDA views the various degrees of similarity.[11] These guidances along with the initial questions and answers response, the description of meeting processes between sponsors and FDA, and the naming approach for biological products have all been published in a final form.[7-11,14] Several guidances remain in draft form including the approach to biosimilar labeling as well as the long-awaited documentation of FDA's approach to biosimilar interchangeability.[16-18] The considerations related to biosimilar interchangeability are important not just from the language of the statute and the related guidance, but also in terms of how we view the clinical equivalence of these medications to branded biologics.

UNDERSTANDING INTERCHANGEABILITY

One of the hallmarks of success for the generics market has been FDA's ability to declare a medication directly equivalent to a branded product while accompanied by state legal statutes allowing pharmacists' substitution without direct prescriber intervention.[19] Attempting to apply a related designation and comparable legal approach to biosimilars is proving to be a challenging and controversial endeavor.[20-22] Substitution of generic medications for their branded counterparts is made easier because these molecules are simple and identical chemical replicas of the originator. Biosimilars are neither simple nor identical copies of branded biologics, as discussed in Chapter 3. In addition, while we can glean some level of understanding about various aspects of biosimilars based on the experience globally, interchangeability is not one of those considerations. Other regulatory bodies, including the European Union, do not designate biosimilars as interchangeable.[6] This aspect of the biosimilar experience will be one on which the U.S. market will have to take the lead.

TABLE 6-3. FDA Biosimilar Guidances[7-18]

Guidance Name	Summary
Scientific considerations in demonstrating biosimilarity to a reference product	■ Introduces FDA's approach to determination of biosimilarity including key concepts such as: ● Use of a stepwise approach in demonstrating biosimilarity ● Totality-of-the-evidence approach ● General scientific principles in conducting comparative structural analyses, functional assays, animal testing, human PK and PD studies, clinical immunogenicity assessments, and comparative clinical studies
Quality considerations in demonstrating biosimilarity of a therapeutic protein product to a reference product	■ Provides recommendations to sponsors on the scientific and technical information for the chemistry, manufacturing, and controls section of a biosimilar application ■ Includes factors critical for assessing similarity of a proposed biosimilar: ● the expression system, manufacturing process, assessment of physicochemical properties, functional activities, receptor binding and immunochemical properties, impurities, reference product and reference standards, finished drug product, and stability
Biosimilars: questions and answers regarding implementation of the Biologics Price Competition and Innovation Act of 2009: Guidance for Industry	■ Provides answers to common questions from sponsors interested in developing proposed biosimilar products and other stakeholders ■ *Addresses key questions:* ● A proposed biosimilar may have a different formulation, delivery device or container closure system than its reference counterpart provided a sponsor can demonstrate no clinically meaningful differences in terms of safety, purity, or potency. ● A biosimilar sponsor can obtain approval for fewer than all routes of administration, fewer than all presentations, and fewer than all conditions of use for which the originator reference product is licensed. ● A sponsor can use comparative animal or clinical data with a non-U.S-licensed originator product to support a biosimilarity determination. ● A biosimilar application can extrapolate clinical data for one indication to support licensing for use in another indication. ● Additional details or pediatric research requirements are included
Formal meetings between the FDA and biosimilar biological product sponsors or applicants	■ Describes the expectations and recommendations for industry regarding the five types of meetings that can occur during a biosimilar development program

(continued)

TABLE 6-3. (Continued)

Guidance Name	Summary
Clinical pharmacology data to support a demonstration of biosimilarity to a reference product	■ Provides direction to assist sponsors with the design and use of clinical pharmacology studies to support a decision that a proposed therapeutic biological product is biosimilar to a reference product ■ Introduces and defines the four assessments that could result from a comparative analytical characterization of a proposed biosimilar: 　● insufficient analytical similarity, analytical similarity with residual uncertainty, tentative analytical similarity, and fingerprint-like analytical similarity
Reference product exclusivity for biological products filed under Section 351(a) of the PHS Act*	■ Describes FDA's current thinking regarding the determination of the date of first licensure of reference originator products ■ Establishes when FDA can accept a biosimilar application and approve a biosimilar
Biosimilars: additional questions and answers regarding implementation of the Biologics Price Competition and Innovation Act of 2009*	■ Provides answers to additional common questions regarding development of proposed biosimilar products ■ Answers questions related to biosimilarity/interchangeability, provisions related to requirement to submit a BLA for a biological product, and exclusivity ■ *Addresses key points:* 　● Biosimilar sponsors should retain samples of biologic products used in clinical pharmacokinetics and/or pharmacodynamic studies used to support a 351(k) application for 5 years.
Nonproprietary Naming of Biological Products Guidance for Industry	■ Introduces the concept of biological products' nonproprietary name to include an FDA-designated suffix ■ Requires suffixes for both originator biologics and biosimilars ■ Requires suffix to be four letters in length and devoid of meaning ■ Establishes concept of core name and proper name 　● Core name = Name adopted by United States Adopted Names (USAN) council 　● Proper name = core name + four letter suffix attached by a hyphen ■ Includes stated purpose to enhance pharmacovigilance, ensure safe use of biological products, and advance appropriate perceptions regarding biological products

(continued)

TABLE 6-3. (Continued)

Guidance Name	Summary
Implementation of the "Deemed to Be a License" Provision of the Biologics Price Competition and Innovation Act of 2009*	■ Describes FDA's approach to migration of biological products previously approved under section 505 of the Federal, Food, Drug, and Cosmetic Act, which will be deemed to be a license under section 351 of the Public Health Services Act on or before March 23, 2020 ■ Include examples of products affected: • hyaluronidase products, imiglucerase products, insulin, insulin mix, and insulin analog products (including aspart, detemir, glargine, glulisine, and lispro), pancrelipase, pegvisomant, somatropin, taliglucerase alfa, velaglucerase alfa, and thyrotropin alfa
Labeling for Biosimilar Products Guidance for Industry*	■ Describes requirements for developing the draft labeling to accompany submission for biosimilar products ■ The biosimilar label can rely on FDA's finding of safety and effectiveness for the reference product in providing the essential scientific information needed to facilitate prescribing; biosimilar applicants should incorporate relevant data and information from the reference product labeling, with appropriate product-specific modifications ■ In general, does not expect biosimilar label to include data from biosimilar clinical trials as studies generally would not be designed to independently demonstrate the product's safety and efficacy, but support demonstration of biosimilarity ■ Provides examples of when the full nonproprietary name (including suffix) should and should not be used ■ Will generally limit indication information to those uses for which the biosimilar is approved ■ Provides that label should include biosimilarity statement identifying the reference product to which the biosimilar is compared
Considerations in Demonstrating Interchangeability with a Reference Product*	■ Describes the type and extent of data and information needed to demonstrate interchangeability. ■ Requires sponsors to conduct a switching study or studies to support interchangeability designation. ■ Establishes expectations for biologics of differing complexity. Less complex biologics with a finger-print like analytical similarity could be designated interchangeable based on a switching study. ■ May require more complicated biologics without a finger-print like characterization to have postmarketing data as well as an appropriately designed switching study. ■ Describes how a sponsor could conduct an integrated study to support both biosimilarity and interchangeability.

(continued)

TABLE 6-3. (Continued)

Guidance Name	Summary
Statistical Approaches to Evaluate Analytical Similarity*	■ This guidance provides direction regarding the statistical analyses used in the analytical characterization of a biosimilar. ■ The FDA recommends the use of a risk-based approach in the analytical similarity assessment of biosimilar quality attributes. This approach should reflect the potential for various quality attributes to impact clinical performance as well as the degree of uncertainty related to those attributes. ■ Tier 1 attributes, those with the highest potential for clinical impact, should be evaluated through statistical equivalence tests. Quality ranges can be applied to tier 2 attributes (those with lower risks) and visual comparisons can be used for tier 3 attributes (those with the lowest risk). ■ Comparisons should include a minimum of 10 lots of the originator reference product and 10 lots of the biosimilar. The reference product lots should account for the originator's variability.

*Guidance in draft format at the time of writing; therefore, could be subject to additional change.

FDA = Food and Drug Administration; PD = pharmacodynamics; PHS = Public Health Service; PK = pharmacokinetics.

Interchangeability—What Does the Legislation Say?

First, we must carefully consider what the interchangeability definition actually implies given the context of existing legislation. According to the BPCI Act, an interchangeable biologic is not only highly similar to the originator reference product, but can be expected to produce the same clinical result in any given patient.[1] Furthermore, this designation also endorses the conclusion that a patient can be switched between an interchangeable biologic and the originator reference product without any greater risk of safety or diminished efficacy than if he or she had remained on the originator product.[1] The interchangeability definition requires additional information beyond that required for a biosimilarity determination.[20]

Second, there are two allowances defined by the BPCI Act for products deemed interchangeable: one that affects the manufacturer and one that impacts the prescriber/pharmacist/patient.[1] For the first product approved as interchangeable to an originator biologic, FDA cannot approve another interchangeable biosimilar to that same molecule for a period of one year.[1] This period of exclusivity is intended to incentivize manufacturers to pursue such a designation. Given the additional requirements and related cost associated with this definition, the extent to which manufacturers consider interchangeability a necessary pursuit remains unknown.[20] The second element of interchangeability has created even more uncertainty, specifically the extent to which this definition will influence the substitution of biosimilars for originator biologics.[21,22] The BPCI Act states that for biologics deemed interchangeable, such products can be substituted for the originator without the intervention of the prescriber.[1] This potential application of the interchangeability concept has drawn the awareness and concern of manufacturers—both biosimilar and originator—pharmacists, physicians, patients, as well as industry and patient advocacy organizations.[21,22] All of these voices have expressed multiple points of view regarding the extent to which biosimilar interchange should receive endorsement or restriction.

Interchangeability—What FDA Requires

The regulatory difficulty in establishing interchangeability has been a key contributor to the uncertainty about this issue.[23] The lack of clarity was moderated with the publication of FDA's draft guidance on the subject.[17] Although there had been some consideration that postmarketing data alone could justify the interchangeability status of biosimilar, FDA has now stated that such information is not a sufficient substitute for a switching study.[17] The required switching study or studies must be of appropriate size, duration, and scope and include enough switches between the biosimilar and the originator reference product to assess potential immune responses and the resulting impact on safety and efficacy.[17] Specifically, the arm in which patients are exposed to both the originator and the reference product should include at least two separate exposure periods to each agent (i.e., three switches).[17] FDA also includes comments for sponsors who wish to conduct an integrated study that would support both a biosimilarity determination as well as assess the impact of switching.[17] In such a circumstance, the sponsor is encouraged to conduct a two-part study between the proposed biosimilar and the originator reference product.[17] After the time period for determination of no clinically meaningful differences, the subjects in the reference arm should be re-randomized either to continue receiving the reference product (non-switching arm) or the proposed biologic (switching arm).[17]

FDA has also suggested two approaches to interchangeability depending on key attributes of a proposed interchangeable biologic.[17] If a product is a less complex biologic, has a low level of immunogenic adverse events, and has been shown to have a meaningful, fingerprint-like analytical similarity, a switching study may be sufficient to justify the interchangeability designation.[17] In contrast, if a biologic has a higher structural complexity, lacks a fingerprint-like analytical similarity, and has a greater likelihood of serious adverse events related to immunogenicity, then such an approach is not appropriate.[17] Instead, the sponsor should first pursue licensure as a biosimilar and collect postmarketing data that when combined with a switching study or studies would support the interchangeability designation.[17] This consideration also elevates a significant concern regarding the perception of interchangeable biologics and non-interchangeable biosimilars.

Interchangeability—What It Is Not

One critically important detail we must understand when discussing the concept of interchangeability is that a biosimilar that has received this designation is not intrinsically superior to a non-interchangeable biosimilar simply as a function of having attained this status.[20] The standard that must be met for biosimilars is that of high similarity based on the totality of the evidence established through analytical characterization, nonclinical, and clinical trials.[1] Interchangeability requires additional evidence provided to establish that switching back and forth between the biosimilar and the originator reference product does not result in a clinically meaningful adverse outcome.[17,20] However, the product that is ultimately deemed as interchangeable is the same biologic originally approved as a non-interchangeable biosimilar.[20] This consideration has prompted some concerns that a biosimilar lacking an interchangeability designation could be considered inferior.[23] As described above, the current draft recommendation is that more complex biologics with a greater potential for immunogenicity-related adverse events and lacking the fingerprint-like analytical similarity should first pursue licensing as a non-inter-changeable biosimilar.[17] If clinicians are hesitant to use these products, it could prove even more difficult to establish a post-marketing track record to support an ultimate data submission for the interchangeability determination.

Interchangeability in Practice

Even with the definitions provided by the BPCI Act and the interchangeability guidance document, a consensus on how interchangeability will affect practice remains elusive. For example, biosimilar manufacturers and the payer community have tended to articulate interchangeability as a mechanism by which biosimilar adoption could be encouraged to promote competition and realize cost savings. For this audience, interchangeability would facilitate substitution where clinically appropriate.[22] Conversely, other groups view less favorably the use of interchangeability to facilitate substitution. Within the prescriber community, this change has been perceived at least by some as a loss of control of a physician's ability to direct patient care.[21] In addition, patient advocacy groups have raised questions about patient safety if a third party (e.g., payer, pharmacist) were to select a biosimilar, particularly one not labeled for interchange, in the absence of a physician's awareness and consent.[21] This concern has led to use of the terminology of non-medical switching to characterize substitution initiated without the direct intervention of the prescriber.[21] These worries also reflect that the broad acceptance of the interchange and substitution of generic medications has not yet translated to the biosimilars market.

Prior to FDA's publication of the interchangeability draft guidance, some switching information was made available in the biosimilar applications approved to date. Sandoz's phase III clinical trial that supported approval of filgrastim-sndz included treatment arms where patients were transitioned between the biosimilar and the originator versions of filgrastim.[24] Even though the evaluation of switching patients between products was not a primary objective of this trial, there were no clinically meaningful differences in the arms where switching occurred as compared to the groups where participants were treated solely with the branded agent or the biosimilar.[24] The evaluation of etanercept-szzs also included a phase where study subjects were alternated between biosimilar and branded therapy.[25] No differences in adverse events were noted.[25] Still, this study was not intended to support a formal request for interchangeability. The approvals for infliximab-dyyb and adalimumab-atto included a single transition from the branded product to the biosimilar to provide insight on the safety of these agents in patients previously exposed to the originator.[26,27] No differences in safety or immunogenicity were reported in these single transitions.[26,27] Still, a single transition is a different intervention than moving a patient back and forth between therapies.

The European Medicines Agency does not make any comments or conclusions regarding interchangeability of biosimilars, but leaves such issues up to individual nations.[28] Thus far, most countries have chosen not to allow nonprescriber-directed interchange of biosimilars for originator products.[29] However, one country, France, has passed legislation allowing pharmacist-directed substitution, provided the physician has not prohibited such an action.[29] A 2012 analysis of clinical trial data, pharmacovigilance databases, and an overview of the published literature revealed no safety issues related to switching involving biosimilars of somatropin, filgrastim, and epoetin.[30] More recently, a much publicized, large Phase IV trial provided additional insight related to a one-time switch from originator to biosimilar infliximab.[31]

The NOR-SWITCH trial, funded by the Norwegian government, was a randomized, noninferiority, double-blind, Phase IV trial of 482 patients who had been stable on branded infliximab for at least 6 months with 52-week follow-up across 40 sites throughout Norway.[31] Patients on stable treatment with originator infliximab were randomized to either remain on the same version or switch to biosimilar infliximab (CT-P13), now approved in the United States as infliximab-dyyb. The diseases treated included Crohn's disease, ulcerative colitis, spondyloarthritis, rheumatoid arthritis, psoriatic arthritis, and chronic plaque psoriasis.[31] Disease worsening occurred in 53 (26%) patients in the infliximab originator group compared with 61 (30%) in the biosimilar group for an adjusted treatment difference of –4.4%, 95% CI –12.7 to 3.9.[30] This difference met the prespecified noninferiority margin of 15%.[31] In addition, the frequency of severe adverse events, overall adverse events, and adverse events leading to discontinuation were similar between groups.[31] This study demonstrates only a single switch and not a continued interchange between originator and biosimilar. In addition, the trial looked at usage across multiple indications.[31] Still, it offers additional documentation of similar performance in a post-marketing setting.

State Legislative Involvement in the Interchangeability Discussion

Although FDA is the ultimate arbiter of which products are deemed as interchangeable, it is up to each state and their pharmacy practice acts to determine how this designation is interpreted and integrated into practice. Even though no interchangeable biosimilars yet exist, multiple states have entertained and even enacted regulations concerning substitution thanks at least in part to the actions of branded biologics' manufacturers.[32] As of October 1, 2017, 35 states and Puerto Rico have enacted such legislation.[33]

Common elements of biosimilar substitution language include the following:[33]

- FDA approval— FDA must approve biological products as interchangeable to be eligible for substitution

- Prescriber authority to prevent substitution—prescribers retain *dispense as written* or *brand medically necessary* authority

- Prescriber and patient notification of substitution—when a substitution occurs, some extent of notification or communication to the prescriber is required; some states have included requirements that patients must be notified and consent to biosimilar substitution

- Records—state legislation usually includes considerations for record retention of substitutions

- Immunity—some state regulations have also included some degree of immunity for pharmacists who make substitutions that are in accordance with state law

- Cost or pricing—some state regulations require the pharmacist to provide the patient with information on the cost or price of the biologic and the biosimilar

Purple Is the New Orange

If FDA ultimately designates a biosimilar as interchangeable, it will be critical to communicate that information to prescribers, pharmacists, and other clinicians. To address this need, FDA has created a unique reference for biologics called the "Purple Book."[34] As the name implies, this resource is intended to occupy a comparable role to the "Orange Book," which lists therapeutic equivalency ratings for generic medications. The Purple Book identifies biosimilars approved for reference products and ultimately will delineate which of those agents possesses an inter-changeability designation.[34] Although limited in content presently, this reference will exert greater meaning as the market continues to expand.

A Different Approach to Interchangeability

After all of this consternation, there is some consideration that interchangeability will ultimately be less impactful within the biosimilar market than the generic environment, primarily given the profile of the originator biologics targeted for competition. Unlike many retail blockbuster prod-ucts, especially those orally delivered, biologic drugs are parenterally administered, either by a healthcare provider or by a well-trained patient.[35,36] As such, these agents are usually managed through a hospital setting, inpatient or outpatient, or provided through the increasingly expanding market of specialty pharmacies.[35,36] In the inpatient or hospital-related outpatient setting, phar-macists will help direct the use of biosimilars through a formulary management approach via the organization's Pharmacy and Therapeutics (P & T) Committee.[5] As such, a preapproved process for biosimilar substitution, with or without a formal interchangeability designation, can occur similar to therapeutic interchange programs. For self-administered products, it is anticipated that biosimilars, like their originator counterparts, will also be managed according to the formulary strategies of pharmacy benefit management organizations, including the use of prior authoriza-tion and step therapy.[37] Therefore, a prescriber will likely have already consented to the use of a biosimilar before a dispensing circumstance occurs. As a result, the impact of the interchange-ability status may be less influential on the actual supply of biosimilars and instead could be interpreted inaccurately as a statement of biosimilar quality. Pharmacists must provide education to guard against this error.

THE REALITY OF THE INTERCHANGEABILITY CONTINUUM

Another important element of the biosimilar experience is not just to what extent biologic drugs can be considered substitutable, but what factors influence our level of comfort with the inter-change of all pharmaceuticals. For example, our default expectation is that small molecules, given their simpler molecular structure, are easily and always substitutable. Yet, we also know that such conclusions are not universally held especially when discussing the use of certain anti-sei-zure medications, immunosuppressants, and anticoagulants, frequently labeled as narrow ther-apeutic index drugs.[38] For some patients and clinicians, the therapeutic equivalency rating is not adequate to alleviate all concerns about identical performance of generic versions of branded molecules. Conversely, both health systems and pharmacy benefit management companies have long refined the success of formulary management to support therapeutic interchange of agents that are not only molecularly distinct, but possess differing doses and frequencies of administration.[5] In addition, we also can reference the interesting example of intravenous immune globulins. Each of these agents is a naturally sourced, distinctly licensed biologic.[39] Still, many of these unique agents are frequently used interchangeably, particularly in times of limited supply.[40] It remains to be seen where biosimilars, both non-interchangeable and interchange-able, fit on this spectrum of equivalence (see **Figure 6-1**).[38,40] If biosimilars, initially approved as non-interchangeable, achieve a significant level of use and acceptance, the return on investment may not justify pursuit of the interchangeability designation. Conversely, if the market continues to develop slowly, this additional level of information gathering may be necessary. We may also discover that the importance of interchangeability varies by molecule.

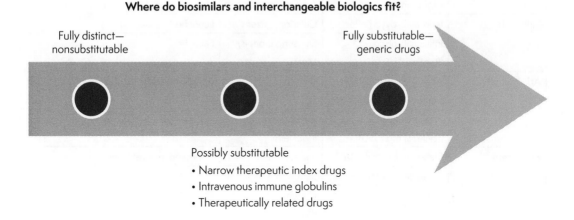

Where do biosimilars and interchangeable biologics fit?

Fully distinct—
nonsubstitutable

Fully substitutable—
generic drugs

Possibly substitutable
• Narrow therapeutic index drugs
• Intravenous immune globulins
• Therapeutically related drugs

FIGURE 6-1. THE CONTINUUM OF SUBSTITUTABILITY.[36-38]

BPCI Act in Action

The increasing number of approved biosimilars continues to shed light on the way in which FDA interprets and implements the provisions of the 351(k) pathway including the use of analytical and clinical data, the approach to indication extrapolation, the bridging of non-U.S. originator data, biosimilar naming, labeling, the use of advisory committee recommendations, and many other circumstances.[25-27,41,42] Each approval represents more opportunities for pharmacists to learn not only about each agent, but about the biosimilar paradigm itself. Given the number of molecules pending in some stage of development (see **Table 6-4**), there will be many more opportunities in the near future to watch the biosimilar pathway grow and evolve.[41-43]

TABLE 6-4. Biosimilars Approved or Presently Pending with FDA[41-43]

Molecule	Drug Name	Sponsor	Status
Filgrastim	Filgrastim-sndz (Zarxio)	Sandoz	Launched
	Filgrastim	Apotex	BLA; initial user fee date passed
	Filgrastim	Adello Biologics	User fee date, May 2018
Infliximab	Infliximab-dyyb (Inflectra)	Celltrion/Pfizer	Launched
	Infliximab-abda (Renflexis)	Samsung Bioepis/ Merck	Launched
Adalimumab	Adalimumab-atto (Amjevita) ABP 501	Amgen	Approved; not yet launched
	Adalimumab-adbm (Cyltezo) BI695501	Boehringer Ingelheim	Approved 8-25-2017
Etanercept	Etanercept-szzs (Erelzi)	Sandoz	Approved; not yet launched
	Etanercept (Brenzys)	Samsung Bioepis	Phase III
	CHS-0214	Coherus Biosciences	Phase III
Bevacizumab	Bevacizumab-awwb (Mvasi) ABP 215	Amgen and Allergan	Approved 9-14-2017
	BI695502	Boehringer Ingelheim	Phase III
	PF-06439535	Pfizer	Phase III
	Biosimilar bevacizumab	Biocon	Phase III
	FK238	Kyowa	Phase III
Trastuzumab	MYL-1401O	Mylan	BLA; user fee date December 2017; positive advisory committee hearing
	CT-P10	Teva and Celltrion	User fee date, March 2018
	Biosimilar trastuzumab	Samsung Bioepis/ Merck	Phase III
	PF-05280014	Pfizer	User fee date, May 2018
Rituximab	CT-P10 (Truxima)	Teva/Celltrion	User fee date, February 2018
	GP2013	Sandoz	User fee date, May 2018
	BI695500	Boehringer Ingelheim	Phase III
	ABP 798	Amgen	Phase III
	PF-05280586	Pfizer	Phase III
Biosimilar pegfilgrastim	MYL-1401H	Mylan and Biocon	BLA; user fee date passed
	Biosimilar pegfilgrastim	Apotex	BLA; user fee date passed
	CHS-1701	Coherus Biosciences	BLA; received complete response letter
	Biosimilar pegfilgrastim	Sandoz	BLA; received complete response letter
Epoetin alfa	Epoetin (Retacrit)	Hospira/Pfizer	BLA; received complete response letter

BLA = biologics license application; FDA = Food and Drug Administration.

KEY POINTS

■ The BPCI Act established the framework for approval of biosimilars and continues to be defined through both guidance publication as well as the demonstration of key principles through actual approvals.

■ The 351(k) approval pathway has similar characteristics to other existing pathways but also has unique attributes that continue to be finalized.

■ The issue of interchangeability remains a controversial consideration not only from the standpoint of regulatory definition, but also in terms of how such a designation might affect prescribing and use of biosimilars.

CONCLUSION

The BPCI Act granted FDA the authority to approve applications for biosimilars as well as further define the framework by which such products have and will continue to receive licensing endorsement. Some aspects of biosimilar regulations are well defined and have been repeatedly demonstrated in the approvals that have already taken place. Others continue to evolve and some still require further definition, most notably interchangeability. Regardless, pharmacists must have a complete understanding of the current status of these elements to interpret the meaning of biosimilar approvals and translate that information for additional stakeholders, including physicians, other clinicians, and patients.

REFERENCES

1. Title VII: Improving access to innovative medical therapies. Subtitle A: Biologic Price Competition and Innovation Act of 2009. www.fda.gov/downloads/drugs/guidancecomplianceregulatoryinformation/ucm216146.pdf (accessed 29 Sept 2017).

2. Carver KH, Elikan J, Lietzan E. An unofficial legislative history of the Biologics Price Competition and Innovation Act of 2009. *Food Drug Law J.* 2010; 65:670-818.

3. FDA Guidance Agenda: New & Revised Draft Guidances CDER Is Planning to Publish During Calendar Year 2017. www.fda.gov/downloads/Drugs/GuidanceComplianceRegulatoryInformation/Guidances/UCM417290.pdf (accessed 29 Sept 2017).

4. BPCIA litigation summary chart. Big Molecule Watch. www.bigmoleculewatch.com/bpcia-litigation-summary-chart/ (accessed 29 Sept 2017).

5. Lucio SD, Stevenson JG, Hoffman JM. Biosimilars: implications for health-system pharmacists. *Am J Health-Syst Pharm.* 2013; 70:2004-17.

6. McCamish M, Woollett G. The state of the art in the development of biosimilars. *Clin Pharmacol Ther.* 2012; 91:405-17.

7. Food and Drug Administration. Guidance for industry. Scientific considerations in demonstrating biosimilarity to a reference product, April 2015. www.fda.gov/downloads/drugs/guidancecomplianceregulatoryinformation/guidances/ucm291128.pdf (accessed 29 Sept. 2017).

8. Food and Drug Administration. Guidance for industry. Quality considerations in demonstrating biosimilarity of a therapeutic protein product to a reference product, April 2015. www.fda.gov/downloads/drugs/guidancecomplianceregulatoryinformation/guidances/ucm291134.pdf (accessed 29 Sept 2017).

9. Food and Drug Administration. Guidance for industry. Biosimilars: Questions and answers regarding implementation of the Biologics Price Competition and Innovation Act of 2009. www.fda.gov/downloads/Drugs/GuidanceComplianceRegulatoryInformation/Guidances/UCM444661.pdf (accessed 29 Sept 2017).

10. Food and Drug Administration. Guidance for industry. Formal meetings between the FDA and biosimilar biological product sponsors or applicants. www.fda.gov/downloads/Drugs/Guidance-ComplianceRegulatoryInformation/Guidances/UCM345649.pdf (accessed 29 Sept 2017).

11. Food and Drug Administration. Guidance for industry. Clinical pharmacology data to support a demonstration of biosimilarity to a reference product, December 2016. www.fda.gov/downloads/Drugs/GuidanceComplianceRegulatoryInformation/Guidances/UCM397017.pdf (accessed 29 Sept 2017).

12. Food and Drug Administration. Guidance for industry, draft guidance. Reference product exclusivity for biological products filed under section 351(a) of the PHS Act. www.fda.gov/downloads/Drugs/GuidanceComplianceRegulatoryInformation/Guidances/UCM407844.pdf (accessed 29 Sept 2017).

13. Food and Drug Administration. Guidance for industry, draft guidance. Biosimilars: additional questions and answers regarding implementation of the Biologics Price Competition and Innovation Act of 2009. www.fda.gov/downloads/Drugs/GuidanceComplianceRegulatoryInformation/Guidances/UCM273001.pdf (accessed 29 Sept 2017).

14. Food and Drug Administration. Guidance for industry. Nonproprietary naming of biological products. http://www.fda.gov/downloads/drugs/guidances/ucm459987.pdf (accessed 29 Sept 2017).

15. Food and Drug Administration. Guidance for industry, draft guidance. Implementation of the "Deemed to be a License" provision of the Biologics Price Competition and Innovation Act of 2009. www.fda.gov/downloads/drugs/guidancecomplianceregulatoryinformation/guidances/ucm490264.pdf (accessed 29 Sept 2017).

16. Food and Drug Administration. Guidance for industry, draft guidance. Labeling for biosimilar products. www.fda.gov/downloads/drugs/guidancecomplianceregulatoryinformation/guidances/ucm493439.pdf (accessed 29 Sept 2017).

17. Food and Drug Administration. Guidance for industry, draft guidance. Considerations in demonstrating interchangeability with a reference product. www.fda.gov/downloads/Drugs/GuidanceComplianceRegulatoryInformation/Guidances/UCM537135.pdf (accessed 29 Sept 2017).

18. Food and Drug Administration. Guidance for industry, draft guidance. Statistical approaches to evaluate analytical similarity. www.fda.gov/downloads/Drugs/GuidanceComplianceRegulatoryInformation/Guidances/UCM576786.pdf (accessed 29 Sept 2017).

19. Boehm G, Yao Lixin, Han Liang, Zheng Q. Development of the generic drug industry in the US after the Hatch-Waxman Act of 1984. *Acta Pharmaceutica Sinica B*. 2013; 3:297-311.

20. McCamish M, Pakulski J, Sattler C, Woollett G. Toward interchangeable biologics. *Clin Pharmacol Ther*. 2015; 97:215-7.

21. Alliance for Safe Biologic Medicines. https://safebiologics.org (accessed 29 Sept 2017).

22. Biosimilars Forum. About the Biosimilars Forum. www.biosimilarsforum.org/ (accessed 29 Sept 2017).

23. Brennan Z. Biosimilar interchangeability: "Careful what you wish for." http://raps.org/Regulatory-Focus/News/2016/09/08/25812/Biosimilar-Interchangeability-%E2%80%98Careful-What-You-Wish-For%E2%80%99/ (accessed Sept. 29, 2017).

24. Blackwell K, Semiglazov V, Krasnozhon D et al. Comparison of EP2006, a filgrastim biosimilar, to the reference: a phase III, randomized, double-blind clinical study in the prevention of severe neutropenia in patients with breast cancer receiving myelosuppresive chemotherapy. *Ann Oncol*. 2015; 26:1948-53.

25. FDA briefing document. Arthritis Advisory Committee Meeting. July 13, 2016. BLA 761042. GP2015, a proposed biosimilar to Enbrel (etanercept). www.fda.gov/downloads/AdvisoryCommittees/CommitteesMeetingMaterials/Drugs/ArthritisAdvisoryCommittee/UCM510493.pdf (accessed 29 Sept 2017).

26. FDA briefing document. Arthritis Advisory Committee Meeting. February 09, 2016. BLA 125544. CT-P13, a proposed biosimilar to Remicade (infliximab), Celltrion. www.fda.gov/downloads/AdvisoryCommittees/CommitteesMeetingMaterials/Drugs/ArthritisAdvisoryCommittee/UCM484859. pdf (accessed 29 Sept 2017).

27. FDA briefing document. Arthritis Advisory Committee Meeting. July 12, 2016. BLA 761024. ABP 501, a proposed biosimilar to Humira (adalimumab), Amgen. www.fda.gov/downloads/AdvisoryCommittees/CommitteesMeetingMaterials/Drugs/ArthritisAdvisoryCommittee/UCM510293.pdf (accessed 29 Sept 2017).

28. Bennett CL, Chen B, Hermanson T et al. Regulatory and clinical considerations for biosimilar oncology drugs. *Lancet Oncol.* 2014; 15:594-605.

29. Thimmaraju PK, Rakshambikai R, Farista R, Juluru K. Legislations on biosimilar interchangeability in the US and the EU—developments far from visibility. www.gabionline.net/Sponsored-Articles/Legislations-on-biosimilar-interchangeability-in-the-US-and-EU-developments-far-from-visibility (accessed 29 Sept 2017).

30. Ebbers HC, Muenzberg M, Schellekens H. The safety of switching between therapeutic proteins. *Exp Opin Biol Ther.* 2012; 12:1473-85.

31. Jorgensen KK, Olsen IC, Goll GL et al. Switching from originator infliximab to biosimilar CT-P13 compared with maintained treatment with originator infliximab (NOR-SWITCH): a 52-week, randomized, double-blind, non-inferiority trial. *Lancet* 2017; 389:2304-16.

32. Silverman E. Controversial biosimilar legislation heats up in California. www.forbes.com/sites/edsilverman/2013/08/22/controversial-biosimilar-legislation-heats-up-in-california/#68c482622242 (accessed 29 Sept 2017).

33. State laws and legislation related to biologic medications and substitution of biosimilars. National Conference of State Legislatures. www.ncsl.org/research/health/state-laws-and-legislation-related-to-biologic-medications-and-substitution-of-biosimilars.aspx (accessed 29 Sept 2017).

34. Food and Drug Administration. Purple Book: Lists of licensed biological products with reference product exclusivity and biosimilarity or interchangeability evaluations. www.fda.gov/drugs/developmentapprovalprocess/howdrugsaredevelopedandapproved/approvalapplications/therapeuticbiologicapplications/biosimilars/ucm411418.htm (accessed 29 Sept 2017).

35. Schumock GT, Li EC, Suda KJ et al. National trends in prescription drug expenditures and projections for 2016. *Am J Health Syst Pharm.* 2016; 73:1058-75.

36. Express Scripts 2015 Drug Trend Report. March 2016. http://lab.express-scripts.com/lab/drug-trend-report (accessed 29 Sept 2017).

37. Falit BP, Singh SC, Brennan TA. Biosimilar competition in the United States: statutory incentives, payers, and pharmacy benefit managers. *Health Aff (Millwood).* 2015; 34:294-301.

38. Pope ND. Generic substitution of narrow therapeutic index drugs. US Pharm. 2009; 34(suppl):12-9. https://www.uspharmacist.com/article/generic-substitution-of-narrow-therapeutic-index-drugs (accessed 29 Sept 2017).

39. FDA. Immune globulins. www.fda.gov/BiologicsBloodVaccines/BloodBloodProducts/ApprovedProducts/LicensedProductsBLAs/FractionatedPlasmaProducts/ucm127589.htm (accessed 29 Sept 2017).

40. ASHP guidelines on medication cost management strategies for hospitals and health systems. *Am J Health Syst Pharm.* 2000; 65:1368-84.

41. Pending biosimilar applications. The Pink Sheet, FDA Performance Tracker (subscription) (accessed 29 Sept 2017).

42. Mullard A. Bracing for the biosimilar wave. *Nat Rev Drug Discov.* 2017; 16:152-4.

43. Drugs@FDA: FDA approved drug products. https://www.accessdata.fda.gov/scripts/cder/daf/ (accessed 29 Sept 2017).

CHAPTER 7

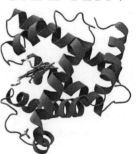

BIOSIMILAR CLINICAL TRIAL REQUIREMENTS

Among the many concepts unique to the biosimilarity paradigm, one of particular significance for pharmacists and other clinicians to internalize is the appropriate role of clinical data in biosimilar approvals. While essential, the clinical information included in a biosimilar application is more targeted as compared to the interrogation of a completely novel molecular entity and focused on a different outcome assessment.[1,2] These differences are made possible by the extensive and robust analytical characterization technologies, nonclinical data, pharmacokinetic (PK) and pharmacodynamic (PD) studies, and immunogenicity analyses that precede Phase III trial information.[1-3] If these successive evaluations reveal a high degree of similarity, the resulting clinical trial (or trials) is focused on any residual uncertainty regarding the safety, purity, and potency of the proposed biosimilar.[1,2] If no such differences are found, the molecule's biosimilarity is confirmed without having to replicate unnecessarily the clinical trials associated with the originator.[1,2] It is these efficiencies that enable the manufacture and marketing of a competing biologic at a lower expense.[1]

If biosimilars are to be accepted, pharmacists must embrace not only the validity of analytical data, as described in Chapter 4, but also this unique approach to clinical information including the importance of PK, PD, and immunogenicity studies. Clinicians must also be fully cognizant and comfortable with the additional principles of indication extrapolation and the use of non-U.S. originator data to support a streamlined and more cost-effective development approach for competing biologics. In this chapter, we will examine these concepts based on the Food and Drug Administration (FDA) guidance documents and the biosimilar approvals that have already taken place.

PRINCIPLES OF BIOSIMILAR CLINICAL TRIAL DESIGN

FDA's Approach to Clinical Trial Information

According to statutory requirements of the Biologics Price Competition and Innovation (BPCI) Act, an application for a biosimilar contains "a clinical study or studies (including the assessment of immunogenicity and pharmacokinetics or pharmacodynamics) that are sufficient to demonstrate safety, purity and potency in 1 or more appropriate conditions of use for which the reference product is licensed and intended to be used."[3] These requirements differentiate approval of biosimilars from that of generics, where no expectations for clinical data exist. The text of the BPCI Act and multiple FDA guidance documents illustrate further the role of clinical data as shown in **Table 7-1**.[4,5]

TABLE 7-1. FDA Guidances Concerning Biosimilar Clinical Trial Data[4,5]

Guidance	Contents
Clinical pharmacology data to support a demonstration of biosimilarity to a reference product	■ Overarching concepts related to clinical pharmacology testing for biosimilar products are introduced ■ Includes recommendations for key elements of pharmacokinetic (PK) and pharmacodynamic (PD) trials such as study (crossover versus parallel) design, study population, dose, route of administration, desired PK and PD measures, defining the appropriate PD time profile, and the statistical comparison of PK and PD results ■ States that selected study population, dose, and route of administration for assessment should be the ones most sensitive in detecting a difference between the biosimilar and the originator reference product ■ Addresses the use of "bridging" data from a non-U.S.- licensed comparator to support a biosimilar application

Scientific considerations in demonstrating biosimilarity to a reference product	■ Describes the critical considerations in demonstrating biosimilarity including a stepwise approach to biosimilar evaluation, embracing the "totality-of-the-evidence" concept, and the general scientific principles in conducting the comparative analytical studies, animal testing, human PK and PD testing, clinical immunogenicity assessments, and comparative clinical trials
	
	■ Expects sponsor to conduct comparative human PK and PD studies (if there are relevant PD measures(s)) and a clinical immunogenicity assessment
	
	   ● A comparative clinical study or studies is required unless there is no residual uncertainty about the biosimilar following the PK, PD, and immunogenicity studies
	
	■ Includes the type and extent of data required for a biosimilarity demonstration:
	
	   ● nature and complexity of the reference product,
	   ● extent to which differences in structure or function predict differences in clinical outcome,
	   ● extent to which human PK or PD data predict clinical outcomes,
	   ● extent of clinical benefit with the reference product,
	   ● extent of any other clinical experience with the proposed product (e.g., if product has been marketed outside the United States)
	
	■ Must have all endpoints, study population, sample size and duration of study to allow for adequate detection of clinically meaningful differences between the biosimilar and the originator product
	
	■ Generally expects the clinical study or studies to establish statistical evidence that the proposed product is neither inferior to the reference product by more than a specified margin nor superior to the reference product by more than a (possibly different) specified margin
	
	■ Allows sponsors to pursue extrapolation of indications across the labeled uses of the originator reference product
	
	■ Allows use of comparative data of biosimilar with a non-U.S.–licensed originator to support approval provided effective bridge can be established

Throughout its guidance documents, FDA repeatedly emphasizes that every aspect of a study—its design, dose and route of administration, indication for evaluation, population investigated, duration, and measures of safety and efficacy—must be justified with the agency.[4,5] Biosimilar sponsors must apply a stepwise approach throughout their product's development with each sequence addressing the remaining residual uncertainties from previous steps in the process.[4,5] If these preceding steps are accomplished successfully, the extent of clinical trial information needed to complete the evaluation should be modest in size and scope. As a result, the preceding analyses including PK, PD, and immunogenicity studies must be well-structured.

The Importance of PK, PD, and Immunogenicity Data

When the words "clinical trial" are invoked, clinicians tend to envision large, Phase III, randomized, double-blind studies, usually focused on establishing superiority of one agent over another intervention in a specific population of patients.[6] However, the FDA-coined phrase "totality of the evidence" is more appropriate for biosimilars.[5] Rather than viewed in isolation, biosimilar clinical information is one of a set of elements needed to establish a high degree of similarity.[1] Information gleaned from each step of development is used to frame the biosimilar's comparability to an originator biologic.[1] Even the clinical data derived from Phase I trials, including those in healthy volunteers, are critically important.[4] The BPCI Act grants FDA the discretion to base a biosimilar approval on the data made available through PK, PD, and immunogenicity studies without requiring the completion of a Phase III trial.[3] Thus far, approved biosimilars have been accompanied by at least one Phase III study.[7-11] However, as the biosimilar model continues to mature, the possibility of resting approval decisions on PK, PD, and immunogenicity data could become increasingly possible.[4] One biosimilar application currently in development for the biologic pegfilgrastim includes no trial data in patients, only PK, PD, and immunogenicity information in healthy volunteers.[12]

Clinical Pharmacology Studies in Action

The utility of PK/PD studies is demonstrated in the approval for filgrastim-sndz, the first biosimilar licensed in the United States.[9] While supported primarily by a Phase III study in breast cancer patients receiving myelosuppressive chemotherapy, the application was supplemented with four PK, PD, and safety studies involving healthy volunteers as shown in **Table 7-2**.[9]

The PK and PD trials for this molecule illustrate critical aspects of biosimilar clinical pharmacology study design. For example, the PK and PD studies were all crossover trials conducted in healthy volunteers who received filgrastim subcutaneously at a varying range of doses.[9] According to FDA guidance, the crossover design is recommended for PK and PD studies where the molecule has a short half-life, a rapid PD response, and generally a lower risk of immunogenicity.[4] Conversely, a parallel design should be used when a molecule has a longer half-life and a greater risk of immunogenicity that could increase with repeated exposure and possibly alter PK and PD results.[4] If it is safe to administer the product to healthy subjects, this population is preferred as there are likely to be fewer confounding effects that could alter PK and PD results.[4] The subcutaneous route of administration is desired, as compared to intravenous dosing, as it is more likely to help identify clinically meaningful differences related to product absorption and immunogenicity.[4] Finally, PK and PD studies may involve lower doses than the standard dose or a range of doses.[4] For some medications, the common and/or higher dose may correlate with the plateau of the dose-response curve, making it more difficult to assess comparability.[4] Lower

TABLE 7-2. Summary of Trials Included in Application for Filgrastim-sndz[9]

Study ID	Design Features	Objectives	Dose/Route/Duration
Studies Comparing Biosimilar to U.S.–licensed Originator Filgrastim			
EP06-109	Randomized double-blind, 2-way crossover in healthy subjects (N = 28)	1. ANC, PK 2. CD34+, safety	10 mcg/kg, sub-Q single dose
EP06-302	Randomized double-blind, active controlled study (N = 204)	1. Safety (incidence of severe adverse events and immunogenicity), efficacy (duration of severe neutropenia) 2. Included a Cycle 1 PK sub-study (N = 54)	5 mcg/kg, sub-Q multiple dose
Studies Using European Approved Originator Filgrastim			
EP06-103	Randomized double-blind, 2-way crossover in HS, with two dose groups (N = 28/dose)	1. ANC 2. PK, CD34+, safety	2.5 and 5 mcg/kg, sub-Q single and multiple (7 day) dose
EP06-105	Randomized, double-blind, 2-way crossover in HS (N = 24)	1. ANC 2. PK, safety	1 mcg/kg, sub-Q single dose
EP06-101	Randomized, double-blind, 2-way crossover in HS (N = 32)	1. PK 2. CD34+, ANC, safety	10 mcg/kg, sub-Q single and multiple (7D) dose

HS = healthy subjects; ANC = absolute neutrophil count; Sub-Q = subcutaneous.

doses or a variety of doses may be used to assess PK and PD metrics on the steeper part of the dose-response curve.[4] A notable benefit for filgrastim is that the evaluation of this molecule is greatly enhanced by the availability of PD markers that are easy to assess and are accepted as measures of efficacy: the absolute neutrophil count (ANC) and CD34+.[9] Such markers will not necessarily be available with all subsequent biosimilars.[4]

In addition to PK and PD, immunogenicity is a critical element of clinical pharmacology studies.[4] Both the choice of patient to study and indication to be assessed are exceedingly important to ensuring the quality of immunogenicity trials.[4] For example, given the molecule and the patient population in which it is used, immunogenicity tends to be less of a concern with filgrastim.[9] However, other biologic products have a greater potential for immune-mediated responses and antibody development, as will be discussed in Chapter 8.[7] One example involves the erythropoietin molecule and its association with the very rare, yet very severe type of immunogenicity called pure red cell aplasia (PRCA).[13] Given this potential immune-related response, an erythropoietin biosimilar sponsor would be expected to include a rigorous investigation of immunogenicity.[13] In the FDA's analysis of the first biosimilar erythropoietin submitted for review, the application included two immunogenicity studies in patients with chronic kidney disease.[14] These study participants would be considered more appropriate for assessment of immunogenicity as compared to oncology patients (i.e., immunosuppressed patients), another population in which erythropoietin can also be used.[4]

Even after all of this preparatory work, most biosimilar approvals will usually require clinical data (i.e., Phase III trial), which will be detailed in this next section.

BIOSIMILAR CLINICAL TRIAL DESIGN

Superiority Is Nice, But Equivalence Will Suffice

In most Phase III clinical trials, the overarching context is usually that of evaluating a novel therapy against either a placebo or previously established treatment.[6] As a result, the focus of the study is to identify the clinical effectiveness of the new treatment and ideally establish its superiority over another intervention.[6] In the biosimilar environment, it is understood that the originator reference product has previously demonstrated evidence of safety and efficacy.[2] Therefore, the comparison of products is to ensure the absence of any clinically meaningful difference between the biosimilar and originator biologic.[2] In contrast to superiority trials, an equivalence study design is usually chosen for biosimilars.[2] In this analysis, investigators, with input from regulators, establish what is described as the minimally clinically important difference (MCID), which can be denoted as δ.[2,6] The MCID is the acceptable difference in outcome where two competing therapies would still be considered clinically similar.[2,6] The MCID is calculated based on information derived from previous clinical trials of the originator biologic against placebo.[6] As shown in **Figure 7-1**, a meta-analysis of randomized trials helps establish the lower confidence interval between the originator and placebo (M1 in the graphic).[6] The sponsor in conjunction with FDA or another regulatory authority agrees to the percent of the treatment effect, usually 50% to 75%, that must be preserved to demonstrate equivalence.[6] That value, in this case M2, is now the MCID, or δ.[6] Variations greater than this limit suggest that two products are in fact not equivalent, thus failing to achieve the standard of biosimilarity. However, if the results of the trial fall into this range, the biosimilar can be considered equivalent. Failure to confirm equivalence can yield numerous other outcomes as shown in **Figure 7-2**.[6] Evidence of inferiority or superiority does not meet the standard of biosimilarity.

MCID—Infliximab As an Example

FDA used five studies to establish the MCID for infliximab-dyyb.[7] The efficacy of originator infliximab (combined with methotrexate) was reflected as an American College of Rheumatology 20 (ACR20) treatment response difference against placebo ranging from 18% to 38% across these trials.[7] A fixed effect, meta-analysis of these studies yielded a difference between originator infliximab and placebo of 28.4%, 95% CI, 23.6% to 33.3%.[7] The specific MCID or similarity margin established was ± 12%, corresponding to approximately 50% of the conservative treatment effect of infliximab as compared to placebo.[7] In the Phase III rheumatoid arthritis (RA) study submitted as part of the application, 60.9% of biosimilar infliximab patients and 58.9% of originator infliximab patients met the ACR20 response rate at week 30.[7] The absolute difference of 2% in treatment response fell within the pre-established confidence interval (90% CI: −4.6%, + 8.7%; 95% CI: −5.8%, +9.9%) and validated the preservation of treatment effect demonstrating the equivalence of the biosimilar to the originator.[7]

Although the equivalence design is generally expected by FDA, there may be some circumstances where ruling out only inferiority is adequate to establish that no clinically meaningful differences exist between the biosimilar and the originator reference product.[2] Thus far, the FDA-licensed biosimilars were all subject to equivalence trials.[7-11]

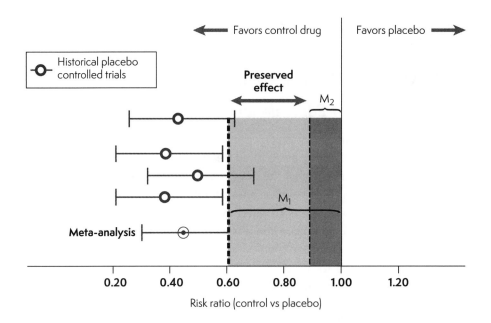

FIGURE 7-1. CALCULATION OF MCID.

Source: Reprinted from Dranitsaris G, Dorward K, Hatzmichael E, Amir E. Clinical trial design in biosimilar drug development. *Invest New Drugs.* 2013;31:479-87 with permission of Springer.

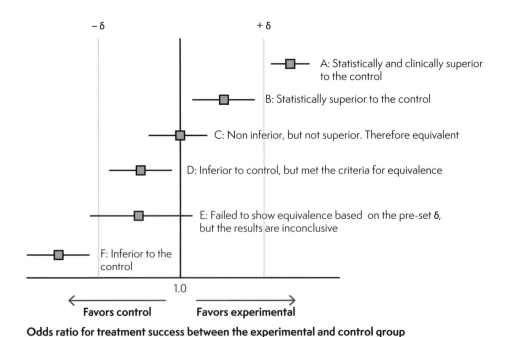

FIGURE 7-2. COMPARING AND CONTRASTING SUPERIORITY AND EQUIVALENCE STUDIES.

Source: Reprinted from Dranitsaris G, Dorward K, Hatzmichael E, Amir E. Clinical trial design in biosimilar drug development. *Invest New Drugs.* 2013; 31:479-87 with permission of Springer.

Management of Missing Data in Biosimilar Trials

Another area where superiority and noninferiority trials differ in biosimilarity discussions is how protocol violations and patient withdrawals are addressed.[6] In superiority trials, the recommended approach is to follow the intention to treat (ITT) standard where all patients are included in the efficacy analysis regardless of whether or not they received treatment.[6] In this circumstance, randomization integrity is maintained and the difference in the treatment effect between the experimental and control group reflects a conservative estimate.[6] However, in an equivalence or noninferiority study, the ITT approach increases the likelihood that a difference in treatments may be missed.[6] As a result, it is recommended that both ITT and per-protocol analyses be conducted for biosimilar trials and any variations further evaluated.[6] FDA may also request additional sensitivity analyses related to the absence of data due to patient withdrawals. For example, in the review of biosimilar adalimumab-atto, a 6% dropout rate was noted in one of the Phase III clinical trials used to support approval.[8] As a result, FDA requested that an evaluation of sensitivity, specifically a tipping point analysis, be conducted.[8] A tipping point analysis is a tool where missing data caused by patient dropout are replaced with values such that a predetermined p value is no longer significant.[15] If the data have to be modified to such an extent that the likelihood of these changes would be considered highly unlikely and/or implausible, the study results are considered robust in spite of missing data.[15] Such was the case with adalimumab-atto where the demonstration of equivalence was preserved throughout the analysis.[8]

MANY FROM ONE: INDICATION EXTRAPOLATION

As listed in Table 7-1, key considerations for biosimilar clinical study design include the determination of the indication that will be studied along with the population to be evaluated, the sample size, and the duration of the trial.[5] All of these elements must be sensitive enough to allow for the detection of clinically meaningful differences between the reference product and the proposed biosimilar.[5] In addition, the choice of indication is critical to the opportunity for extrapolation.[5]

FDA possesses the authority to extrapolate clinical data from the use of a biosimilar in one specific circumstance to support approval across other indications.[5] This capability enables further efficiency in eliminating the requirement for a biosimilar applicant to conduct clinical trials in all indications for which licensing is sought. FDA has stated in its guidance that extrapolation must be scientifically justified.[5] Thus far the strategy of biosimilar applicants has been to seek licensing across all eligible (i.e., non-orphan) indications of the originator reference product.[7-11]

According to FDA, extrapolation is based on information such as the following:

- The mechanism of action in each condition for which licensure is sought
- The PK and bio-distribution of the product in different patient populations
- The immunogenicity of the product in different patient populations
- Differences in expected toxicities in each condition of use and patient population
- Any other factor that may affect the safety or efficacy of the product in each condition of use and patient population for which licensure is sought[5]

Extrapolation creates several considerations. First, the indication in which a biosimilar is studied should be sensitive enough to detect clinically meaningful differences that would be relevant to the multiple uses of the originator product.[5] That use may not necessarily be the initial indication in which the originator was first licensed or even the circumstance in which it is most commonly prescribed.[7-11]

The selection of indications for study and its impact on extrapolation of indications have already resulted in controversy for some of the initial biosimilar applications evaluated by the FDA and other regulatory agencies.[7,8,16,17] One such example involves infliximab-dyyb.[7,16,17] Originator infliximab is used in multiple patient populations (e.g., rheumatoid arthritis and related conditions versus inflammatory bowel diseases) in which the proposed mechanism of action possibly could vary across the different disease states, although the data remain inconclusive.[7] As such, accepting the evidence of clinical utility in one patient group as support for approval in other indications has proven challenging for different regulators.[16] In the example of infliximab-dyyb, the sponsor investigated the product in RA and ankylosing spondylitis (AS).[7] However, there was no initial evaluation in inflammatory bowel diseases (IBD) (see Chapter 4 for more information).[7,8] In spite of the plausible differences in mechanisms of action, FDA concluded that the totality of the evidence across all of the information submitted for approval justified licensing of the biosimilar not only for the RA-related uses, but also the IBD indications.[7] The European Medicines Agency also chose to license the Celltrion product in all of the indications of the originator while Health Canada initially limited approval to the populations in which it was investigated and similar patient groups.[16] Health Canada has since granted biosimilar infliximab full indication coverage including labeling for the IBD based on additional data provided by the manufacturer.[17] If the concept of extrapolation has proven challenging for regulatory agencies to understand and implement, the degree of difficulty will likely prove even greater in actual practice circumstances.

Extrapolation: What It Means

When considering extrapolation, we must not lose sight of a critical concept regarding this practice. Extrapolation is not the application of safety and efficacy evidence of the biosimilar as demonstrated in one use to support the licensing of that same product in other indications.[18] Instead, extrapolation occurs between the originator and the biosimilar (**Figure 7-3**).[18] If comparative clinical trial information in an appropriately selected, sensitive indication coupled with the preceding analytical and nonclinical data have demonstrated that no differences exist between the biosimilar and the originator in terms of safety, purity, and potency, it is scientifically justified to endorse the proposed biosimilar for the other uses in which the branded product is licensed.[18] Extrapolation of indications has been consistently applied in U.S. biosimilar approvals.[7-11] In some cases, this concept has been more easily adopted as in the example of filgrastim and etanercept, where the mechanisms of action are considered more consistent across uses.[9,10] Pharmacists must educate physicians on the scientific justification of extrapolation as more products enter the market.

Although extrapolation can be substantiated scientifically, the likelihood of obtaining full labeling can vary by product as sponsors have the discretion to seek only certain indications in their filing.[19] If a biosimilar sponsor does not perceive all indications equally useful to a robust market acceptance of their product, they could pursue only one or a subset of indications for which the originator has labeling.[19] Also, remaining orphan exclusivities for newer indications of the originator may prevent a complete mirroring by the biosimilar, at least upon initial

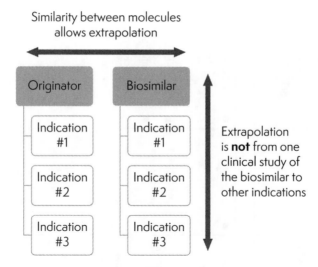

FIGURE 7-3. UNDERSTANDING EXTRAPOLATION.[18]

approval.[7-9,11] **Table 7-3** lists the indications for the currently approved biosimilars as well as the uses not presently included in the labeling of these products.[7-11,20-28]

LIKE A BRIDGE OVER GLOBAL WATERS

In addition to extrapolation, the other highly significant efficiency that can support the approval of a biosimilar is the ability to use data generated from trials involving non-U.S.-licensed originator products.[5,19] It is not surprising that blockbuster originator molecules are commonly prescribed in markets beyond the United States.[29] Suppliers investing in biosimilars would benefit from the opportunity to license their versions of these molecules across different regions of the globe.[25] If sponsors were required to replicate trials comparing their biosimilars to the versions of the originator reference products licensed in each nation, this duplication of clinical data would further increase costs and limit potential savings.[29] The ease and expense of conducting clinical trials for biosimilars also varies across countries.[30] In more developed nations with a higher access to healthcare, it may prove challenging to recruit patients for a trial in which the desired outcome is that the biosimilar under investigation will be shown to work the same as a preexisting treatment.[30] As a result, the most economical process would be to conduct one or as few trials as possible to support approval across multiple countries. To address this need, FDA allows the use of non-U.S.-licensed originator data in support of biosimilar approval provided a scientifically justified "bridge" can be developed.[5,19]

We will illustrate this example by reviewing the approval of infliximab-dyyb.[7] Infliximab-dyyb was licensed based on among other things, data from two randomized, double blind, parallel group clinical trials: a Phase III study in RA patients (PLANETRA) and a Phase I study in AS subjects (PLANETAS).[31,32] The active comparator in these studies was the European version of originator infliximab.[31,32] Both the PLANETRA and PLANETAS studies demonstrated comparability between biosimilar and European originator infliximab in terms of efficacy, safety, PK, and immunogenicity.[7,31,32] However, as all biologics vary, the applicability of these data to U.S.-licensed originator infliximab was not immediately established. As a result, Celltrion also

TABLE 7-3. Indication Coverage for Currently Approved Biosimilars[7-11,20-28]

Filgrastim-sndz (Zarxio)	Infliximab-dyyb (Inflectra)	Etanercept-szzs (Erelzi)	Adalimumab-atto (Amjevita)	Infliximab-abda (Renflexis)	Adalimumab-adbm (Cyltezo)	Bevacizumab-awwb (Mvasi)
Directly Studied						
■ Cancer patients receiving myelosuppressive chemotherapy*	■ Rheumatoid arthritis (in combination with methotrexate) ■ Ankylosing spondylitis	■ Plaque Psoriasis**	■ Rheumatoid Arthritis* ■ Plaque psoriasis	■ Rheumatoid arthritis (in combination with methotrexate)	■ Rheumatoid arthritis*	■ Non-squamous non-small cell lung cancer (NSCLC)
Extrapolated						
■ Patients with acute myeloid leukemia receiving induction or consolidation chemotherapy ■ Cancer patients receiving bone marrow transplant ■ Patients undergoing peripheral blood progenitor cell collection and therapy ■ Patients with severe chronic neutropenia	■ Psoriatic arthritis ■ Plaque psoriasis ■ Crohn's Disease* ■ Pediatric Crohn's disease ■ Ulcerative colitis	■ Rheumatoid Arthritis* ■ Polyarticular Juvenile Idiopathic Arthritis ■ Psoriatic Arthritis** ■ Ankylosing Spondylitis	■ Juvenile Idiopathic Arthritis (patients 4 years of age and older) ■ Psoriatic Arthritis ■ Ankylosing spondylitis ■ Adult Crohn's disease ■ Ulcerative colitis	■ Psoriatic Arthritis ■ Plaque Psoriasis ■ Crohn's Disease* ■ Pediatric Crohn's Disease ■ Ulcerative Colitis ■ Ankylosing Spondylitis	■ Juvenile Idiopathic Arthritis (patients 4 years of age and older) ■ Psoriatic Arthritis ■ Ankylosing spondylitis ■ Adult Crohn's Disease ■ Ulcerative Colitis	■ Metastatic colorectal cancer* ■ Glioblastoma ■ Metastatic renal cell carcinoma ■ Cervical cancer

(continued)

TABLE 7-3. (Continued)

Filgrastim-sndz (Zarxio)	Infliximab-dyyb (Inflectra)	Etanercept-szzs (Erelzi)	Adalimumab-atto (Amjevita)	Infliximab-abda (Renflexis)	Adalimumab-adbm (Cyltezo)	Bevacizumab-awwb (Mvasi)
			Indications Not Covered			
■ Patients acutely exposed to myelosuppressive doses of radiation***	■ Pediatric Ulcerative Colitis***	■ None	■ Treatment of Uveitis*** ■ Treatment of Hidradenitis Suppurativa*** ■ Juvenile idiopathic arthritis 2 years to 4 years of age*** ■ Crohn's Disease (pediatric)***	■ Pediatric Ulcerative Colitis Disease	■ Treatment of Uveitis*** ■ Treatment of Hidradenitis Suppurativa*** ■ Juvenile idiopathic arthritis 2 years to 4 years of age*** ■ Crohn's Disease (pediatric)***	■ Platinum-resistant epithelial ovarian, fallopian tube, or primary peritoneal cancer ■ Platinum-sensitive epithelial ovarian, fallopian, or primary peritoneal cancer

*Initial indication in which originator approved.

**Sandoz recently requested deletion of these indications from the label; but change not due to safety or efficacy issues.

***Orphan indication.

conducted a randomized, double blind, parallel group, single dose study in healthy volunteers (see **Table 7-4**) comparing biosimilar infliximab to both the U.S. and European version of origi-nator infliximab.[7] This study demonstrated comparable PK, safety, and immunogenicity across all three products establishing the bridge.[7] As the biosimilar performed in a highly similar fashion to both versions of originator infliximab (U.S. and European Union [EU]), the results of PLANETRA and PLANETAS could be adopted as evidence of biosimilarity for infliximab-dyyb as compared to U.S.-licensed originator product.[7] **Tables** 7-4, **7-5**, **7-6**, and **7-7** illustrate the clinical trial structure, including bridging studies, used to support biosimilarity determinations for inflixi-mab-dyyb, etanercept-szzs, adalimumab-atto, and infliximab-abda.[7,8,10,11]

Although the approval of filgrastim-sndz did not involve a formal bridge, data from trials involving the biosimilar compared to the EU-approved originator product were utilized as supporting information.[9]

It should be noted that the approaches to bridging trials will vary by molecule as well as upon each supplier's interaction with FDA. An example of that variation can be seen with the approval for adalimumab-atto.[8] Amgen in its application conducted two clinical trials, one comparing their biosimilar to the U.S. version of originator adalimumab in RA patients and one comparing their product to European originator adalimumab in plaque psoriasis patients.[8] Given the use of non-U.S.-labeled adalimumab, Amgen established a bridge in 203 healthy subjects comparing the European and U.S. version of the originator and their biosimilar.[8] Amgen conducted these trials even though the RA study was the only one FDA requested.[33] Nevertheless, the study data involving European originator product were used to support the licensing of adalimumab-atto.

Extrapolation and bridging of data of non-U.S.-licensed products will continue to be essen-tial aspects of the biosimilar approval methodology as both principles allow for the efficiency and decreased costs needed to enable competition for branded biologics. The extent to which both strategies are used and the necessary amount of confirmatory information to allow their use will vary by molecule.[7-11,27] Nevertheless as we look to future biosimilar products, we can see both strategies in use for the development of additional competing agents.

One such example includes Amgen's biosimilar version of bevacizumab. Amgen conducted a Phase III, randomized, double-blind, comparative clinical study of their biosimilar ABP215 against EU-approved bevacizumab in 642 patients with metastatic or recurrent non-squamous, non-small cell lung cancer (NSCLC).[27] This trial was used to support licensing in the NSCLC use as well as five other indications (i.e., non-orphan) for which the originator product is licensed, including metastatic colorectal cancer, glioblastoma multiforme, metastatic renal cell carci-noma, and cervical cancer.[27] **Table 7-8** shows the trials supporting the approval of biosimilar bevacizumab.[27]

WILL CLINICAL DATA ALWAYS BE ENOUGH?

As we have seen, it is possible to develop a clinical program that supports approval of a biosim-ilar across multiple indications using targeted data, extrapolation of indications, and bridging of data to non-U.S. licensed products.[7-11,27] However, it remains to be seen if this degree of infor-mation will be sufficient to support actual use in the clinical practice settings, particularly when the biosimilars in question are intended for the treatment of high acuity disease states such as the oncology-related indications. The biosimilars initially approved have either been supportive

TABLE 7-4. Summary of Clinical Studies to Support Infliximab-dyyb Approval[7]

Study (Dates)	Design	Objectives	Subjects	Treatments	Endpoints
Controlled Studies in Patients					
CT-P13 3.1 (Global, ex-U.S.) 54 weeks (12/10–07/12)	R, DB, PG comparative clinical study: efficacy, safety, PK, immunogenicity	Efficacy, safety, PK, immunogenicity	Moderate to severe RA, MTX-IR N = 606	CT-P13 3 mg/kg + MTX EU-approved infliximab 3 mg/kg	ACR 20
CT-P13 1.1 (Global, ex-U.S.) 54 weeks (12/10–07/12)	R, DB, PG PK, efficacy, safety, immunogenicity	PK, efficacy, safety, immunogenicity	Moderate to severe AS N = 250	CT-P13 5 mg/kg EU-approved infliximab 5 mg/kg	ASAS20
Controlled Study in Healthy Volunteers					
CT-P13 1.4 Single Dose (10/13–07/13)	R, DB, PG, SD 3-way PK bridging	PK, safety, immunogenicity	Healthy volunteers N = 213	CT-P13 5 mg/kg EU-approved infliximab 5 mg/kg US-licensed infliximab 5 mg/kg	C_{max} $AUC_{0\rightarrow t}$ $AUC_{0\rightarrow inf}$
Extension Studies					
CT-P13 3.2 (~1 year) (02/12–02/14)	OLE	Safety, immunogenicity	RA, Enrolled from controlled study CT-P13 3.1 N = 302	CT-P13 maintenance CT-P13 transitioned from EU-approved infliximab	Adverse event incidence Immunogenicity
CT-P13 1.3 (~1 year) (03/12–06/13)	OLE	Safety, immunogenicity	AS, Enrolled from controlled study CT-P13 1.1 N = 174	CT-P13 maintenance CT-P13 transitioned from EU-approved infliximab	Adverse event incidence Immunogenicity

ACR = American College of Rheumatology; AS = ankylosing spondylitis; ASAS = Assessment of SpondyloArthritis International Society; $AUC_{0\rightarrow t}$ = area under the plasma concentration time curve to the last measured concentration; $AUC_{0\rightarrow inf}$ = area under the plasma concentration time curve extrapolated to infinity; C_{max} = maximum drug concentration; CT-P13 = biosimilar infliximab; DB = double-blind; EU = European Union; IR = inadequate responder; MTX = methotrexate; OLE = open label extension; PG = parallel group; PK = pharmacokinetics; R = randomized; RA = rheumatoid arthritis.

TABLE 7-5. Summary of Clinical Studies to Support Adalimumab-atto Approval[8]

Study	Objective	Design	Subjects	Treatments	Endpoints
PK Similarity Study					
20110217 07/12–10/12	3-way PK similarity, safety, immunogenicity	R, PG, SD, 3-way PK bridging	203 Healthy subjects	40 mg sub-Q: ■ ABP 501 ■ U.S.-adalimumab ■ EU-adalimumab	C_{max} $AUC_{0\to t}$ $AUC_{0\to inf}$
Comparative Clinical Studies					
20120262 07/12–10/12	Efficacy, safety, immunogenicity in RA	26 weeks, R, DB, PG	526 Patients with RA	40 mg sub-Q Q2W + MTX ■ ABP 501 ■ U.S.-adalimumab	ACR 20
20120263 10/13–03/15	Efficacy, safety, immunogenicity in PsO	R, DB, PG Re-randomized at week 16 to either continue EU-Humira or transition to ABP 501	350 Patients with PsO	80 mg sub-Q Day 1, then 40 mg sub-Q Q2W from Wk2: ■ ABP 501 ■ EU-adalimumab	Percent improvement in PASI (secondary = PASI 75, sPGA, BSA)

ABP 501 = biosimilar adalimumab; ACR = American College of Rheumatology; $AUC_{0\to t}$ = area under the plasma concentration time curve to the last measured concentration; $AUC_{0\to inf}$ = area under the plasma concentration time curve extrapolated to infinity; BSA = body surface area; C_{max} = maximum drug concentration; DB: double-blind; EU = European Union; MTX: methotrexate; PASI = Psoriasis Area Severity Index; PG = parallel group; PsO = plaque psoriasis; Q2W = every 2 weeks; R = randomized; RA = rheumatoid arthritis; SD = single dose; sPGA = static Physician's global Assessment; sub-Q = subcutaneous.

care products (i.e., filgrastim) or the tumor necrosis factor alpha inhibitors.[7-11] Although used in the oncology care environment, filgrastim is a less complex biologic that benefits from its rapid onset of action, well-accepted PD markers, and absence of safety issues of severe concern (i.e., immunogenicity).[9] However, additional biosimilars for oncology conditions have either recently received licensure, bevacizumab-awwb, Amgen and Allergan, or are nearing final approval, MYL-1401O, a version of trastuzumab from Mylan and Biocon.[27,34,35] As stated above, the application for ABP 215 included a Phase III trial in NSCLC patients.[27] The data from a Phase III trial comparing originator trastuzumab and MYL-1401O was recently published in the clinical literature and submitted as part of the review process.[36,37] The trial in question demonstrated an equivalent response between the biosimilar and originator in ERBB2-positive metastatic breast cancer patients using the Response Evaluation Criteria in Solid Tumors version 1.1 criteria.[36,37] The trial also showed no differences between products for the secondary outcome measures of time-to-tumor progression, progression-free survival, or overall survival.[36] The results would appear to demonstrate biosimilarity in the breast cancer indication. However, within an accompanying editorial to the published results, the question was posed as to whether these data would suffice in convincing regulators and prescribers to use the biosimilar in ERBB-2 gastric cancer.[38] To

TABLE 7-6. Summary of Clinical Trials for Etanercept-szzs[10]

Study ID	Design	Objectives	Subjects	Treatments	Endpoints
Clinical Pharmacology Studies					
Study 101	R, DB, 2-way cross-over	PK, safety, and immunogenicity	57 healthy subjects	SD 50 m sub-Q: ■ GP2015 ■ EU-Enbrel	C_{max}, AUC_t, and AUC_{inf}
Study 102	R, DB, 2-way, cross-over	PK, safety, and immunogenicity	54 healthy subjects	SD 50 mg sub-Q: ■ GP2015 ■ US-Enbrel	C_{max}, AUC_t, and AUC_{inf}
Study 104	R, DB, 2-way cross-over	PK, safety, and immunogenicity	54 healthy males	SD 50 mg sub-Q: ■ GP2015 ■ EU-Enbrel	C_{max}, AUC_t, and AUC_{inf}
Report 105	A cross-study comparison of studies 101 and 102 (to establish bridge between EU and U.S. Enbrel)				
Comparative Clinical Study					
Study 302	R, DB, PG TP1 (Wk 0-12)	Efficacy, safety, immunogenicity, PK	531 PsO patients	50 mg sub-Q twice weekly: ■ GP2015 ■ EU-etanercept	PASI 75
	R, DB, PG TP2 (switching) (Wk 12–30)	Safety, immunogenicity, PK	PsO patients re-randomized	50 mg sub-Q: weekly GP2015 cont GP2015 switch EU-etanercept cont EU-etanercept switch	Safety, immunogenicity

AUC = area under the curve; DB = double-blind; EU = European Union; GP2015 = biosimilar etanercept; PASI = psoriasis area severity index; PG = parallel group; PK = pharmacokinetic; PsO = plaque psoriasis; R = randomized; sub-Q = subcutaneous; TP = treatment period; Wk = week.

some extent, this consideration may be delayed as the gastric cancer indication still has orphan drug exclusivity, and this use was not pursued upon initial licensing of Mylan's trastuzumab.[37] However, at some point, orphan exclusivity will expire and Mylan could pursue this indication with FDA. If licensing is granted, practitioners will be confronted with the reality of this circumstance.[37] From a scientific standpoint, demonstration of biosimilarity in one indication can be used to support approval for licensing in other uses.[18] Translating that scientific concept into environments such as the oncology setting will necessitate substantial education and reinforcement.

CLINICAL DATA REQUIREMENTS FOR BIOSIMILARITY VS. INTERCHANGEABILITY

The biosimilar approvals that have occurred thus far have provided tremendous insight as to how FDA's guidance documents manifest in actual practice for biosimilarity determinations.[7-11,27,37]

TABLE 7-7. Summary of Clinical Studies to Support Infliximab-abda[11]

Protocol	Objectives	Duration	Subjects	Sample Size	Treatment Arms
SB2-G11-NHV	R, SB, PG, SD 3-way PK bridging	Single dose	Healthy volunteers	N = 159 (53/ arm) 1:1:1 5 mg/kg	SB2 EU-Remicade U.S.-Remicade
SB2-G31-RA	R, DB, PG, Comparative clinical study	54 weeks	RA patients (MTX–IR)	N = 584 1:1 3 mg/kg	■ SB2+MTX (n = 291) ■ EU-Remicade + MTX (n = 293)
	Transition-Extension Period				
	R, DB, Safety and Immunogenicity	24 weeks (weeks 54–78)	RA patients rolled over from part 1 of the study	N = 396 1:1	■ SB2 maintenance (SB2→SB2) (n = 201) ■ EU-Remicade Maintenance (EU-Remi→Eu-Remi) (n = 101) ■ Transition group (EU-Remi→SB2) (n = 94)

DB = double blind; EU = European Union; IR = inadequate responders; MTX = methotrexate; PG = parallel group; PK = pharmacokinetics; R = randomized; SB = single blind; SB2 = biosimilar infliximab; SD = single dose.

However, with the draft interchangeability guidance now available, it is important to understand how clinical trial data supporting interchangeability may vary from that required to establish a non-interchangeable biosimilar.[39]

As described in Chapter 6, a non-interchangeable biosimilar is not inherently inferior to one that is interchangeable.[18] It is simply that additional data are available to demonstrate that switching between the originator and the interchangeable biologic does not result in a greater incidence of adverse outcomes than if the patient had remained solely on the reference product.[18,39]

Like non-interchangeable biosimilars, FDA reiterates in its interchangeability guidance that it recommends a stepwise approach and will apply the totality of the evidence in evaluating a proposed product.[39] **Table 7-9** summarizes some of the differences articulated in the interchangeability guidance.[39]

The interchangeability guidance articulates that a trial to establish the safety of switching treatments would necessarily have to involve the migration of a patient back and forth between the interchangeable biologic and the originator reference product.[39] In addition, unlike biosimilar studies where bridging to non-U.S.-licensed originator product is acceptable, FDA currently states that true interchangeability trials should involve the biosimilar compared against the

TABLE 7-8. Clinical Trials for ABP215, Biosimilar Bevacizumab-awwb[27]

Study	Design	Objectives	Subjects	Treatments	Endpoints
Controlled Study in Patients					
20120265	R, DB, PG PK, Efficacy, Safety, Immunogenicity	PK, efficacy, safety, immunogenicity	Metastatic or recurrent non-squamous NSCLC patients N = 642 (1:1)	ABP215 15 mg/kg EU-approved bevacizumab 15 mg/kg Administered as an IV infusion every three weeks in combination with carboplatin and paclitaxel for 6 cycles	ORR per RECIST v1.1
Controlled Study in Healthy Volunteers					
20110216	R, SB, PG, SD 3-way PK bridging	PK, safety	Healthy volunteers N = 204 (1:1:1)	ABP215 3 mg/kg EU-approved bevacizumab 3 mg/kg U.S.-licensed bevacizumab 3 mg/kg	C_{max} $AUC_{0 \to t}$ $AUC_{0 \to inf}$

ABP215 = biosimilar bevacizumab; EU = European Union; DB = double blind; IV = intravenous; NSCLC = non-small cell lung cancer; ORR = overall response rate; PG = parallel group, PK = pharmacokinetics, R = randomized, RECIST = response evaluation criteria in solid tumors; SB = single blind, SD = single dose.

U.S.-licensed version of the originator product.[39] It should be noted that the guidance currently establishes two processes to obtain an interchangeability designation depending on certain characteristics of the proposed biosimilar.[39] If the agent in question is a less complex molecule, possesses a lower likelihood of immunogenic events, and is characterized with fingerprint-like similarity, it may be possible to conduct one study to achieve the interchangeable biologic designation.[39] Conversely, more complex products with higher incidences of immunogenic events would first have to obtain designation as a non-interchangeable biosimilar and subsequently seek interchangeability approval.[39] Given the recent introduction of this guidance, no trial has yet been completed implementing this approach.

Switching Studies to Date

The Phase III safety and efficacy trial for filgrastim-sndz provides one example on what a switching study might consider.[9] In this double-blind, parallel group study, breast cancer patients

TABLE 7-9. Unique Criteria for Interchangeable Biologics (per FDA Draft Guidance)[5,39]

Issue	Comment
Pursuit of indication coverage	■ Although previous guidances articulated that the sponsor has the discretion of pursuing all or only a subset of indications of the originator, the interchangeability guidance recommends applicants pursue all uses of the reference product
Pursuit of interchangeability on initial licensing	■ This new guidance describes a process by which interchangeability could be achieved based on a switching study depending on a product's complexity, likelihood of having substantial immunogenic adverse events, and extent to which it can be characterized analytically with fingerprint-like similarity ● Products that do not possess these qualities should pursue biosimilarity first, then supplement post-marketing data with a switching study or studies to support a subsequent interchangeability designation
Use of non-U.S. licensed data to support application	■ Although previous guidances and biosimilar approvals have included and allowed non-U.S.-licensed data if an appropriate bridge can be established, switching studies should be conducted against U.S.-labeled originator reference product
Considerations of presentation influence on interchangeability	■ The guidance describes the analysis that will be required to ensure that the presentation(s) of the proposed biologic itself does not prevent the determination of interchangeability.

were randomized to receive the biosimilar or U.S.-originator filgrastim.[9] As seen in **Table 7-10**, patients were randomized into four treatment arms, two of which received the biosimilar in cycle 1 and two of which received the originator in cycle 1.[9] In the following cycles, one of the biosimilar arms was alternated between the biosimilar and the originator.[9] Similarly, in one originator arm, the patients were switched back and forth between the originator and biosimilar.[9]

The primary safety and efficacy analyses were based on cycle 1 exposure, which again demonstrated a highly similar outcome.[9] However, a safety analysis was conducted over all of the cycles and reflected no difference in the numbers of adverse events attributable to filgrastim-sndz as compared with originator filgrastim.[9] Sandoz did not pursue an interchangeability designation, and there was no consideration of conferring such approval on this biosimilar. The Phase III clinical trial supporting etanercept-szzs also included a treatment period where study subjects were switched between European-originator product and the proposed biosimilar at six-week

TABLE 7-10. Treatment Arms for Biosimilar Filgrastim-sndz (EP06-302)[9]

Arm	Number of Patients	Cycle 1	Cycle 2	Cycle 3	Cycle 4	Cycle 5	Cycle 6
1	48	Biosimilar	Biosimilar	Biosimilar	Biosimilar	Biosimilar	Biosimilar
2	48	Biosimilar	Originator	Biosimilar	Originator	Biosimilar	Originator
3	48	Originator	Biosimilar	Originator	Biosimilar	Originator	Biosimilar
4	48	Originator	Originator	Originator	Originator	Originator	Originator

intervals.[10] This study period of the trial was designed to assess safety and immunogenicity.[10] There was no greater incidence of adverse events in patients who were switched between therapies and those who remained on the originator product.[10] However, no interchangeability designation was pursued.[10]

Single Switch Only

Of the other biosimilar approvals, infliximab-dyyb, adalimumab-atto, and infliximab-abda have included data related to a single switch in transitioning patients receiving the originator product to the proposed biosimilar.[7,8,11] For these products, the transition of a non-naïve patient receiving originator product to the biosimilar did not result in any clinically significant differences in terms of safety or immunogenicity.[7,8,11]

WHAT DOES THIS MEAN FOR PHARMACISTS?

Biosimilar clinical trial information represents an interesting paradox. On the one hand, its presence is essential to the biosimilar application process. Yet, it is not meant to stand alone or serve as the only source of validation for biosimilarity.[1,2] Pharmacists and physicians must be cognizant of the principles that guide the construction of clinical trials including indication selection, extrapolation considerations, and the use of bridging. Still, investing significant time in re-evaluating clinical trial data after FDA has endorsed licensing of a biosimilar is likely to be of limited value as the studies in question only confirm comparability. This perspective is reinforced by the approach FDA has taken toward the labeling of biosimilars.[40] In its guidance on the subject, FDA states that approved labeling for the reference product "may be relied on to provide healthcare practitioners with the essential scientific information needed to facilitate prescribing decisions for the proposed biosimilar product's labeled conditions of use."[40] As a result, the package insert for biosimilars will include a "description of the clinical data that supported safety and efficacy of the reference product" as described in the "FDA-approved product labeling for the reference product."[40] If FDA has concluded that the reference product's clinical trial information is sufficient to guide prescribing of the biosimilar, rigorous review of the biosimilar applicant's clinical study information is likely to elucidate limited additional insight. Given the youth of the U.S. biosimilars market, we have yet to reach a threshold of complete comfort and acceptance with that approach.

KEY POINTS

- Clinical trial information is intended to confirm the similarity of the biosimilar to the originator product, not re-establish the relationship between mechanism of action and clinical performance.

- Additional approvals and FDA guidance publication continue to clarify additional aspects of the biosimilar clinical trial experience including the role and use of Phase I data, indication extrapolation, and bridging of non-U.S.-originator data.

- Pharmacists must understand these concepts and educate stakeholders, especially prescribers, as additional biosimilars near approval, particularly those for oncology conditions.

CONCLUSION

Clinical trial data are by no means unimportant within the context of biosimilar review and adoption. Based on statutory requirements, they are an essential element of the approval process. However, their size, scope, and purpose vary from that of a novel originator molecule. This approach is markedly different for clinicians and will take time to embrace. As a result, pharmacists will need to increase their understanding of the regulatory expectations and scientific justifications that validate this approach to support acceptance and educate prescribers and other clinicians. Pharmacists should utilize the licensing of every biosimilar, independent of the actual timing of product launch, to increase their understanding and that of other clinicians regarding these concepts.

REFERENCES

1. McCamish M, Woollett G. The continuum of comparability extends to biosimilarity: how much is enough and what clinical data are necessary? *Clin Pharmacol Ther.* 2013; 93:315-7.

2. Bui LA, Taylor C. Developing clinical trials for biosimilars. *Semin Oncol.* 2014; 41:S15-25.

3. Title VII: Improving access to innovative medical therapies. Subtitle A: Biologic Price Competition and Innovation provisions of the Patient Protection and Affordable Care Act (PPACA). www.fda.gov/downloads/Drugs/GuidanceComplianceRegulatoryInformation/ucm216146.pdf (accessed 27 July, 2017).

4. Food and Drug Administration. Guidance for industry. Clinical pharmacology data to support a demonstration of biosimilarity to a reference product, December 2016. www.fda.gov/downloads/Drugs/GuidanceComplianceRegulatoryInformation/Guidances/UCM397017.pdf (accessed 27 July, 2017).

5. Food and Drug Administration. Guidance for industry. Scientific considerations in demonstrating biosimilarity to a reference product, April 2015. www.fda.gov/downloads/drugs/guidancecomplianceregulatoryinformation/guidances/ucm291128.pdf (accessed 27 July, 2017).

6. Dranitsaris G, Dorward K, Hatzmichael E, Amir E. Clinical trial design in biosimilar drug development. *Invest New Drugs.* 2013; 31:479-87.

7. FDA briefing document. Arthritis Advisory Committee Meeting. February 09, 2016. BLA 125544. CT-P13, a proposed biosimilar to Remicade® (infliximab), Celltrion. www.fda.gov/downloads/AdvisoryCommittees/CommitteesMeetingMaterials/Drugs/ArthritisAdvisoryCommittee/UCM484859.pdf (accessed 27 July, 2017).

8. FDA briefing document. Arthritis Advisory Committee Meeting. July 12, 2016. BLA 761024. ABP 501, a proposed biosimilar to Humira (adalimumab), Amgen. www.fda.gov/downloads/AdvisoryCommittees/CommitteesMeetingMaterials/Drugs/ArthritisAdvisoryCommittee/UCM510293.pdf (accessed 27 July, 2017).

9. FDA briefing document. Oncologic Drugs Advisory Committee Meeting. January 7, 2015. BLA 125553. EP2006, a proposed biosimilar to Neupogen (filgrastim) Sandoz Inc., a Novartis company. www.fda.gov/downloads/AdvisoryCommittees/CommitteesMeetingMaterials/Drugs/OncologicDrugsAdvisoryCommittee/UCM428780.pdf (accessed 27 July, 2017).

10. FDA briefing document. Arthritis Advisory Committee Meeting. July 13, 2016. BLA 761042. GP2015, a proposed biosimilar to Enbrel (etanercept) Sandoz. www.fda.gov/downloads/AdvisoryCommittees/CommitteesMeetingMaterials/Drugs/ArthritisAdvisoryCommittee/UCM510493.pdf (accessed 27 July, 2017).

11. FDA clinical review document. Division of Pulmonary, Allergy, and Rheumatology products. BLA 761054. www.fda.gov/downloads/Drugs/DevelopmentApprovalProcess/DevelopmentResources/UCM557884.pdf (accessed 27 July, 2017).

12. Sutter S. Neulasta biosimilar from Coherus needs better immunogenicity assay after stumble at US FDA. *The Pink Sheet*, June 12, 2017 (subscription).

13. McKoy JM, Stonecash RE, Cournoyer D et al. Epoetin-associated pure red cell aplasia: past, present, and future considerations. *Transfusion.* 2008; 48:1754-62.

14. FDA briefing document. Oncologic Drugs Advisory Committee Meeting. May 25, 2017. BLA 125545. "Epoetin Hospira," a proposed biosimilar to Epogen/Procrit (epoetin alfa). www.fda.gov/downloads/AdvisoryCommittees/CommitteesMeetingMaterials/Drugs/OncologicDrugsAdvisory-Committee/UCM559967.pdf (accessed 27 July, 2017).

15. Yan X, Lee S, Li N. Missing data handling methods in medical device clinical trials. *J Biopharm Stat.* 2009; 19:1085-98.

16. Feagan BG, Choquette D, Ghosh S et al. The challenge of indication extrapolation for infliximab biosimilars. *Biologicals.* 2014; 42:177-83.

17. Health Canada. Regulatory decision summary INFLECTRA. http://www.hc-sc.gc.ca/dhp-mps/prodpharma/rds-sdr/index-eng.php (accessed 27 July, 2017).

18. McCamish M, Pakulski J, Sattler C, Woollett G. Toward interchangeable biologics. *Clin Pharmacol Ther.* 2015; 97:215-7.

19. Food and Drug Administration. Guidance for industry. Biosimilars: Questions and answers regarding implementation of the Biologics Price Competition and Innovation Act of 2009. www.fda.gov/downloads/Drugs/GuidanceComplianceRegulatoryInformation/Guidances/UCM444661.pdf (accessed 27 July, 2017).

20. Zarxio (filgrastim-sndz) package insert. Princeton, NJ: Sandoz Inc; April 2016.

21. Inflectra (infliximab-dyyb) package insert. Celltrion: Yeonsu-gu, Incheon; April 2016.

22. Erelzi (etanercept-szzs) package insert. Princeton, NJ: Sandoz Inc; 2018 January.

23. Amjevita (adalimumab-atto) package insert. Thousand Oaks, CA: Amgen; September 2016.

24. Renflexis (infliximab-abda) package insert. Yeonsu-gu, Incheon: Samsung Bioepsis; April 2017.

25. GaBi OnLine. Boehringer Ingelheim's adalimumab biosimilar "equivalent" to Humira http://gabionline.net/Biosimilars/Research/Boehringer-Ingelheim-s-adalimumab-biosimilar-equivalent-to-Humira (accessed 3 Oct. 2017).

26. Cyltezo (adalimumab-abdm) package insert. Ridgefield, CT: Boehringer Ingelheim Pharmaceuticals, Inc; August 2017.

27. FDA briefing document. Oncologic Drugs Advisory Committee Meeting. July 13, 2017. BLA 761028. ABP215, a proposed biosimilar to Avastin (bevacizumab), Amgen Inc. https://www.fda.gov/downloads/AdvisoryCommittees/CommitteesMeetingMaterials/Drugs/OncologicDrugsAdvisoryCommittee/UCM566365.pdf. (accessed 3 Oct. 2017).

28. Mvasi (bevacizumab-awb) package insert. Thousand Oaks, CA: Amgen, Inc; September 2017.

29. Casey D. Key strategic factors for stakeholders in the current global biosimilar market. *Drug Discov Today.* 2016; 21:208-11.

30. Rompas S, Goss T, Amanuel S et al. Demonstrating value for biosimilars: a conceptual framework. *Am Health Drug Benefits.* 2015; 8:129-39.

31. Yoo DH, Prodanovic N, Jaworski J et al. A phase III randomized study to evaluate the efficacy and safety of CT-P13 compared with reference infliximab in patients with active rheumatoid arthritis: 54-week results from the PLANETRA study. *Arthritis Res Ther.* 2016; 18:82.

32. Park W, Yoo DH, Jaworksi J et al. Comparable long-term efficacy, as assessed by patient-reported outcomes, safety and pharmacokinetics, of CT-P13 and reference infliximab in patients with ankylosing spondylitis: 54-week results from the randomized, parallel-group PLANETAS study. *Arthritis Res Ther.* 2016; 18:25.

33. Sutter S. Biosimilar sponsors may be going overboard on clinical data, FDA says. *The Pink Sheet*, July 13, 2016.

34. Amgen press release. Amgen and Allergan submit biosimilar biologics license application for ABP 215 to U.S. Food and Drug Administration. www.amgen.com/media/news-releases/2016/11/amgen-and-allergan-submit-biosimilar-biologics-license-application-for-abp-215-to-u-s--food-and-drug-administration/ (accessed 3 Oct. 2017).

35. Han DH. Trastuzumab biosimilar BLA submitted to FDA. www.renalandurologynews.com/drugs-in-the-pipeline/trastuzumab-biosimilar-bla-submitted-to-fda/article/571587/ (accessed 3 Oct. 2017).

36. Rugo HS, Barve A, Waller CF et al. Effect of a proposed trastuzumab biosimilar compared with trastuzumab on overall response rate in patients with ERBB2 (HER2)-positive metastatic breast cancer: a randomized clinical trial. *JAMA.* 2017; 317:37-47.

37. FDA briefing document. Oncologic Drugs Advisory Committee Meeting. July 13, 2017. BLA 761074. MYL-1401O, a proposed biosimilar to Herceptin (trastuzumab), Mylan Pharmaceuticals. https://www.fda.gov/downloads/AdvisoryCommittees/CommitteesMeetingMaterials/Drugs/OncologicDrugsAdvisoryCommittee/UCM566369.pdf. (accessed 3 Oct. 2017).

38. Burstein HJ, Scraq D. Biosimilar therapy for ERBB2 (HER2)–positive breast cancer: close enough? *JAMA.* 2017; 317:30-2.

39. Food and Drug Administration. Guidance for industry, draft guidance. Considerations in demonstrating interchangeability with a reference product. www.fda.gov/downloads/Drugs/GuidanceComplianceRegulatoryInformation/Guidances/UCM537135.pdf (accessed 3 Oct. 2017).

40. Food and Drug Administration. Guidance for industry, draft guidance. Labeling for biosimilar products. https://www.fda.gov/downloads/Drugs/GuidanceComplianceRegulatoryInformation/Guidances/UCM493439.pdf (accessed 3 Oct. 2017).

CHAPTER 8

IMMUNOGENICITY AND PHARMACOVIGILANCE IN THE BIOSIMILAR ERA

Most conversations about biosimilars usually include a discussion regarding the relative safety profile of these medications, especially the potential for immune-mediated responses.[1] Such considerations are not particularly surprising given the fact that biosimilars represent a new drug category with which practitioners have limited familiarity.[1] In addition, biosimilars undergo a more rigorous evaluation of safety and efficacy than generic small molecule medications due to their size and complexity.[1] This requirement could create the perception that a greater frequency of adverse events may be anticipated.[1] Clinicians' perspectives may also be influenced by the examples in the clinical literature where biologic adverse events, including those immunogenic in nature, have occurred with follow-on biologics from less-regulated countries as well as with originator products following manufacturing changes.[1-3] Without additional context, this combination of limited or poorly understood information could be viewed as a surrogate warning about the immunogenicity potential of biosimilars now entering the U.S. market.

This chapter is intended to provide a perspective on adverse event considerations of all biologics as well as the requirements of the biosimilars approval process that are structured to ensure comparable safety. We will also describe the need for improved pharmacovigilance in healthcare for all products, small molecule and biologic, originator or follow-on (i.e., generic or biosimilar).[1,4] Such an appreciation will help pharmacists, other practitioners, and by extension patients, avoid unnecessary apprehension regarding the use of biosimilars while continuing to promote safe and effective management of these agents.

BIOLOGIC ADVERSE EVENTS

Although the adverse reaction potential of biosimilars definitely merits the attention of our pharmacovigilance systems, we must keep the discussion framed within a proper context. All biologics, originators and biosimilars, have the capacity to generate adverse events including those immunogenic in nature.[5,6] Due to this fact, the biosimilar approval process mandates that these agents demonstrate similar "safety, purity, and potency" as compared to the originator reference product.[7] Only after a rigorous evaluation, including analyses of safety, can the Food and Drug Administration (FDA) license a biosimilar for approval. As an approved *highly similar* product, the type and frequency of adverse events for a biosimilar would be expected to be the same as the originator reference biologic.[8] The FDA has reiterated and reinforced this expectation in its guidance documents as evidenced in the recently announced approach to biosimilar labeling.[9] Appropriate pharmacovigilance of biosimilars is essential to the safe use of these products just at it has been with originator biologic drugs.[1]

Another important aspect to consider regarding biologic safety is the fact that immune-mediated responses are only one of the pathways by which adverse events can occur, as illustrated in **Figure 8-1** and described in **Table 8-1**.[10,11-15] Our attention to immunogenic responses is heightened because these large, complex globular structures possess an intrinsic capacity to elicit an immune response, unlike small molecule medications, which must bind to a carrier protein before recognition by the immune system.[5] Even with this distinction between types of products, our ability to anticipate the incidence of a specific immune-related adverse event is difficult due to the fact that the cause and resulting impact of immunogenicity can vary greatly.[16,17] No particular property of a protein is an obvious predictor of immunogenicity in humans.[16,17]

Multiple mechanisms contribute to the adverse event profile for every biologic drug.[10] In some circumstances, the mechanism of toxicity is an extension of the biologic's pharmacological activity, both expected events as well as those that are unanticipated.[10] Within the category of nonpharmacological events, both immune- and nonimmune-mediated responses, such as acute phase reactions, can occur.[10] Although most immune responses do not result in any clinically significant effects, severe cases can be life threatening.[5]

Common concerns with biologics cover the spectrum from acute infusion or injection site reactions, to serum sickness, or even the generation of antibodies against the biologic therapeutic and endogenous proteins.[16] Most approved biologics have the capacity to cause anti-

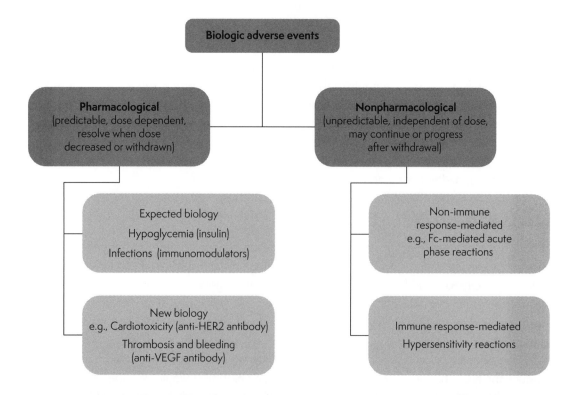

FIGURE 8-1. TYPES OF BIOLOGIC ADVERSE EVENTS.[10,11]

Source: Reprinted from Clarke JB. Mechanisms of adverse drug reactions to biologics. In: *Adverse Drug Reactions, Handbook of Experimental Pharmacology.* J. Uetrecht (ed.). Springer-Verlag Berlin Heidelberg 2010:452-474 with permission of Springer.

TABLE 8-1. Common Adverse Reactions Associated with Biologic Drugs[10-15]

Nonproprietary Name	Example Indications	Adverse Reactions
Adalimumab	Rheumatoid arthritis, Crohn's disease	Infection, neurological events, lymphoma, hypersensitivity, injection site reactions
Bevacizumab	Colorectal cancer	Gastrointestinal perforations, wound healing inhibition, hemorrhage, hypertension, protein urea, infusion reactions
Epoetin alfa	Anemia	Infection, hypertension, cardiovascular events, hypertension, seizures, pure red cell aplasia
Etanercept	Rheumatoid arthritis	Serious infections, malignancies, hepatotoxicity, hypersensitivity, injection site reactions
Infliximab	Rheumatoid arthritis, Crohn's disease	Infection, neurological events, lymphoma, hypersensitivity, infusion reactions
Pegfilgrastim	Neutropenia	Splenic rupture, respiratory distress
Rituximab	Non-Hodgkin's lymphoma, Rheumatoid arthritis	Fever, infusion reactions, tumor lysis syndrome, infections, progressive multifocal leukoencephalopathy
Trastuzumab	Breast cancer, gastric cancer	Cardiomyopathy, hypersensitivity

Source: Adapted with permission from Clarke JB. Mechanisms of adverse drug reactions to biologics. In: Adverse Drug Reactions, Handbook of Experimental Pharmacology. J. Uetrecht (ed.). Springer-Verlag Berlin Heidelberg 2010:452-474. Used with permission from Springer and JB Clarke.

drug antibody (ADA) formation, but their presence does not necessarily affect clinical safety and efficacy.[16] Still, toxicity and/or diminished efficacy are potential outcomes of biologic therapy and, therefore, necessitate a thorough evaluation of any related product, such as a biosimilar.[8]

FOCUS ON IMMUNOGENICITY

The factors that may be involved in the immunogenicity of a biotherapeutic used in humans can generally be characterized as either patient related, treatment related, or associated with the product itself.[16] Factors related to treatment route, patient disease status, and frequency of administration have a complex impact on the clinical immunological response.[16] Among the common routes of administration, the probability of an immune response is generally highest after subcutaneous injection, followed by intramuscular, intranasal, and intravenous routes.[16] Subcutaneous administration localizes and prolongs the exposure of the protein to a small area within close proximity of the lymph nodes where B cells and T cells are present.[16] Lymphatic uptake can enhance exposure to antigen presenting cells.[16] Dendritic cells may potentially be activated if adjuvant-like factors such as impurities, host cell proteins, or endotoxins are present.[16] The type of disease plays a role in the generation of a treatment-related immune response, likely influenced by the patient's immune status.[16] Patients with weak or compromised immune systems or those on immunosuppressive therapy are less likely to develop ADAs than those who are immunocompetent.[16] Short-term therapy is less likely to be immunogenic than long-term therapy, although intermittent treatment is more likely to elicit a response than continuous therapy.[16] Lower doses are generally more immunogenic than higher doses, a characteristic probably related to the phenomenon that the immune system is generally less tolerant of low-abundance proteins.[16]

Within the environment of biosimilars, the patient populations in which the product is used and the overall attributes of dose, route, frequency, and duration of treatment are expected to be the same as that of the originator reference biologic.[7] Therefore, the evaluation of safety must focus on the product-related factors as these elements could potentially vary between originator biologics and biosimilars.[18] As a result, any biosimilar program must examine safety throughout the totality of the development process, from analytical characterization through pharmacokinetic, pharmacodynamic, and clinical efficacy studies continuing to post-marketing monitoring as required.[8]

THE EPREX LEGACY

Much of the heightened wariness regarding biosimilar safety could be traced to various events involving the manufacturing and use of epoetin in Europe during the late 1990s and early 2000s.[3,19] In 1998, physicians in Europe began to identify a substantial increase in the incidence of an extremely rare immune disease, pure red cell aplasia (PRCA).[3,19] PRCA is a very uncommon disorder of erythropoiesis, which results in a progressively worsening, severe, isolated anemia, with a sudden onset.[3] In up to half of cases, there is no identifiable cause and PRCA has been reported even in a patient never exposed to epoetin.[20] Administration of epoetin can result in PRCA through the development of anti-epoetin antibodies that bind and neutralize exogenously-administered as well as endogenously-produced erythropoietin.[3,19,20]

Mad Cow Disease and Biologics

Prior to 1998, there were only three cases of PRCA reported in the literature after epoetin administration.[3] Between January 1998 and July 2003, 195 cases of antibody-mediated PRCA were documented in patients receiving subcutaneous doses of a specific product, epoetin alfa (Eprex; Johnson & Johnson), a version of epoetin not marketed in the United States.[20] The timing of the outbreak seemed to coincide with a manufacturing change of this product.[3,19,20] In 1998, Johnson & Johnson modified the Eprex formulation by removing the human serum albumin stabilizer and replacing it with polysorbate 80 (PS80).[3,19,20] This change was made due to a request of the European Medicines Agency to remove human-derived protein from the formulation to avoid any potential contamination by viruses or prions, which could theoretically lead to Creutzfeldt-Jakob disease, the human manifestation of what is known as Mad Cow disease.[3,19-21] In the almost 20 years since this outbreak was first identified, many mechanisms have been proposed as contributing factors to these events including an increasing trend toward more subcutaneous administration of epoetin, lack of environmental control in product storage, and the modification of the stabilizer.[20] It is this last consideration that has drawn the most attention. Specifically, researchers have suggested that the replacement of human serum albumin with PS80 coupled with the use of an uncoated rubber stopper in Eprex syringes allowed certain leachates to be released from the stopper thus increasing the immunogenicity potential for this drug.[19,20] Regardless of the ultimate cause, multiple corrective actions were taken including restricting Eprex administration to the intravenous route in chronic kidney disease patients, reinforcing appropriate handling procedures for the drug, and replacing the rubber stoppers with ones that were Teflon-coated.[22] Following these changes, the rate of PRCA returned to previous levels and has remained similarly low.[19,22]

In addition to the Eprex example, we have seen other reports of PRCA with epoetin products.[2,23] In 2011, an outbreak of PRCA due to the use of a follow-on version of epoetin was documented in Thailand.[2,23] Researchers identified 30 patients receiving these versions of epoetin who developed a sudden loss of efficacy.[2] Follow-up analysis revealed that 23 of these patients had anti-epoetin antibodies, thus confirming the PRCA diagnosis.[2,23] Also, in a randomized clinical trial of one of the two versions of biosimilar epoetin approved in Europe, two patients were confirmed as having PRCA following receipt of subcutaneous doses of the product, HX575.[23] A root-cause analysis suggested that the incidence of PRCA was associated with tungsten contamination of the prefilled syringe formulation used in the clinical study.[23] In a post-marketing study of 1,700 chronic kidney disease patients receiving HX575, no additional cases of PRCA were reported following intravenous administration of the product.[23]

Were These Actual Examples of Biosimilar Immunogenicity?

The above examples are commonly cited in commentary related to biosimilars and biologic manufacturing.[22,23] While it is true that the need to provide appropriate pharmacovigilance for biosimilars is necessary, the degree of risk is not inherently greater than with originator biologics.[1] For example, Eprex was not and is not a biosimilar, but a fully licensed, branded originator product.[1] Therefore, manufacturing changes for all biologics, originator or biosimilar, must be closely vetted. In addition, the term *biosimilar* does not reflect a universal approach to evaluation and licensing across all countries. Although described as biosimilars, the products used in the Thailand outbreak were biologics from developing countries and were vetted only according to bioequivalence standards of generic molecules.[2,23,24] These products did not undergo the rigorous clinical and immunogenicity assessments that are demanded for biosimilar approval in highly regulated markets like the United States and the European Union.[23,24] In the absence of this degree of evaluation, the outbreak occurred.[24] Finally, the European reports of PRCA with biosimilar epoetin (HX575) were associated with a clinical study product, where a likely contaminant was identified.[25] Management of the production of syringes to eliminate contaminants along with labeling to limit product administration in chronic kidney disease patients only to the intravenous route have mitigated this issue.[26] Furthermore, given continued review of clinical trial data, HX575 received European approval for subcutaneous administration in April 2016.[27] Therefore, biologic drugs, biosimilars included, can result in immunogenic events.[1] In highly regulated markets with thorough biosimilar approval processes, these risks can be minimized and mitigated to ensure comparable safety outcomes as compared to the originator.

In addition to epoetin, antibody development has been noted with other biosimilars approved in Europe.[16] During the clinical development of somatropin (Omnitrope; Sandoz), currently regulated as a small molecule in the United States, the product was found to result in almost 60% of patients developing anti-growth hormone (anti-GH) antibodies.[16] These anti-GH antibodies were not neutralizing and did not impact the efficacy of the product.[16] Subsequent improvement in purification steps helped remove the residual host cell proteins that had previously remained in the formulation so that the rate of antibody development is now consistent with other marketed products.[16] **Table 8-2** lists the antibody formation rate and resulting impact for some commonly used biologics.[5,12-14,28]

This table also illustrates both the importance and challenge of monitoring immune-mediated reactions. In certain circumstances, such as PRCA with epoetin, the incidence is very small,

TABLE 8-2. Examples of Clinically Important Antibodies to Biologic Agents[5,29-33,47]

Product	Antibody Formation (%)	Consequence
Erythropoietin	<1	Pure red cell aplasia
Growth hormone	1–2	No significant effects
Adalimumab	0–54	Lower efficacy rate
Infliximab	0–83	Loss of efficacy, infusion reactions, anaphylaxis
Etanercept	0–13	No known effect (non-neutralizing antibodies)
Rituximab	0–21	Effects unknown

but the potential consequences are extremely significant.[5] For drugs such as infliximab, the rate of antibody formation can vary widely across disease states treated and based on concomitantly administered immunosuppressants.[5,12] These variables should be considered when comparing performance of a biosimilar to the branded originator product.

U.S. licensed biosimilars all include rigorous and detailed evaluations of immunogenicity in both animal and human subjects.[29-33] These analyses have shown that the proposed biosimilars have demonstrated a comparable immunogenicity profile in comparison to their originator counterparts.[29-33] Specifically, in the first biosimilar application accepted by FDA for epoetin alfa, the proposed biosimilar was vetted for immunogenicity, including PRCA, in two randomized clinical trials involving chronic kidney disease patients.[34] In one study, patients were administered biosimilar epoetin intravenously and in the other, the subcutaneous route was used.[34] The rates of antibody drug formation were the same for the biosimilar and the originator product. In addition, no neutralizing antibodies and no instances of PRCA were identified.[34]

REGULATORY EVALUATION OF SAFETY AND IMMUNOGENICITY

Given the potential for adverse reactions, including immune-mediated responses in biologics, the regulatory approval process for biosimilars is very much focused on ensuring comparable safety as compared to originator products. As discussed in Chapter 6, the FDA's expectations for analytical evaluation of safety are described in its guidance document, "Quality Considerations in Demonstrating Biosimilarity of a Therapeutic Protein Product to a Reference Product."[35] In addition, FDA has also described its expectations for the clinical safety assessment of biosimilars in its companion guidance, "Scientific Considerations in Demonstrating Biosimilarity to a Reference Product."[8] According to FDA, "at least one clinical study that includes a comparison of the immunogenicity of the proposed product to that of the reference product will be expected."[8] FDA encourages sponsors to "collect immunogenicity data in any clinical study" where feasible, including human pharmacokinetics or pharmacodynamics trials.[8]

FDA also notes that the assessment of immunogenicity should consider the nature and incidence of immune responses, the clinical relevance and severity of these outcomes, and the populations studied.[8] A comparative parallel design (i.e., head-to-head study) in treatment-naïve patients will usually be required as this structure provides the greatest sensitivity in premarketing assessment of immunogenicity risk.[8] FDA states that the selection of clinical endpoints "associated with immune responses to therapeutic protein products" should consider "the immuno-genicity issues that have emerged during the use of the reference product."[8] Also, the duration of evaluation should consider the course for the generation of immune responses and expected clinical sequelae, the time course for disappearance of the immune responses and clinical sequelae following cessation of therapy, and the length of the product's administration.[8] FDA also directly addresses the antibody parameter that should be assessed in the clinical immuno-genicity assessment.[8] Biosimilar sponsors should evaluate antibody "titer, specificity, relevant isotype distribution, time course of development, persistence, disappearance, impact on phar-macokinetics, and association with clinical sequelae" along with the extent to which product activity is neutralized.[8]

For a biosimilar to receive final licensing by FDA, a demonstration of comparable efficacy and safety is required throughout the development and approval process. In addition, FDA may require additional clinical studies following approval.[8] Furthermore, as with all pharmaceuticals, biosimilars just like originator biologics must be monitored for adverse events through effective post-marketing surveillance.[8] Although we would not expect any greater incidence of negative clinical outcomes with biosimilars, we should improve our pharmacovigilance overall. The next section deals with biosimilar pharmacovigilance considerations beginning with something we take for granted in the generic landscape, the sharing of nonproprietary names with the origi-nator branded product.

BIOLOGIC PHARMACOVIGILANCE—WHAT'S IN A NAME?

One of the more controversial aspects of the biosimilar narrative, against the backdrop of many other complex issues, has been the extent to which these competing products will or will not share the nonproprietary (a.k.a. generic) name of the originator reference product. In the generic medication era, the sharing of the nonproprietary name and the therapeutic equivalency rating have further conveyed the direct link between products.[36] However, whereas generic drugs can be considered identical versions of their brand, the same does not apply to biosimilars.[37] One related concern has been that the use of the exact same, nonproprietary name could inappro-priately imply that a biosimilar is identical to its reference counterpart.[37] Other opinions have conversely suggested that use of the same nonproprietary name of biologics for biosimilar is justified as this process has worked in the more advanced markets of Europe.[37] In addition, branded products following manufacturing changes and comparability determination possess the same nonproprietary name even though they are not identical to the pre-change version (as described in Chapter 3).[38]

Beyond concerns about the misperception of biosimilars as identical molecules, the ability to monitor, identify, and discern adverse events for biosimilars from those of the originator has also generated concern.[1,37] Current estimates and analyses suggest that the accuracy and consistency of adverse drug event documentation for all products, small molecule or biologic, could be substantially improved.[39] One publication postulates that as few as 6% of all adverse drug events are in fact documented.[40] In addition, when adverse event information is captured, it may not provide adequate detail or enable differentiation between related products.[39] Analyses have shown that following the introduction of generic versions of originator small molecules, the majority of adverse events are still reported using the branded name of the reference product rather than assigned to the competitors entering the market.[41] These findings have increased the concern that the capacity to distinguish adverse events between originator biologics and biosimilars may not be adequate to support appropriate pharmacovigilance.[41]

Currently, there are several attributes that could allow for identification of a product down to the level of the batch from which it was derived.[42] Those attributes include the brand name, nonproprietary name, national drug code (NDC) number, and lot number.[42] Unfortunately, a great deal of variation exists throughout patient treatment areas where biologic drugs are administered and/or dispensed.[42] In some higher acuity areas, the capture of the NDC number may be facilitated if bedside barcode scanning is present, while in many nonacute settings, information may still be transcribed manually.[42] Even if some level of product identification is captured, it usually does not extend to the lot number.[39]

As demonstrated in Europe, biosimilars tend to possess unique branded names of their own, unlike generic medications.[43] This distinguishing factor would appear to provide another attribute to differentiate the originator product and any subsequently launched biosimilar. However, brand names can change and many healthcare organizations have adopted the approach of primarily using the non-proprietary name in practice.[44,45] As a result, conversation has focused on whether or not the biologic nonproprietary name (i.e., generic name) should be modified to differentiate between originator medications and biosimilars.[37,44]

Although the global regulatory bodies of FDA and the World Health Organization (WHO) have weighed in with proposed processes, neither appears to have resolved this situation to everyone's satisfaction.[45,46] FDA's approach to naming of both biosimilars and originator biologics is described below.[45]

What's Good for the Biosimilar Is Good for the Originator

FDA's decision, while controversial, at least attempts to address the concerns of both the originator and biosimilar audiences. Although FDA has defined a unique nonproprietary naming structure for biologic drugs, the intent is that the same requirements will ultimately apply to both biosimilars as well as their originator reference counterparts.[45] The central aspect of this naming convention is modifying the nonproprietary names of biologic drugs to include a hyphenated suffix of four lowercase letters that are unique and intentionally devoid of meaning.[45]

In its guidance, FDA has created the concept of *core* and *proper* names.[45] The *core* name for biologics is the adopted name designated by the United States Adopted Names (USAN) council.[45] The *core name* would be what most clinicians would consider the generic or nonproprietary name. Under FDA's defined approach, this core name will be modified with a FDA-designated four-letter suffix to form a biologic's proper name.[45] FDA allows manufacturers to submit a list of 10 proposed suffixes in the order of preference at the time of application submission.[45]

FDA has determined that suffixes should not be promotional, include abbreviations commonly used in clinical practice, contain or suggest any drug substance name, look similar to a currently marketed product, resemble the manufacturer's name, or be too similar to any other product's designated suffix.[45] In addition to the guidance on this naming convention, FDA has also published a proposed rule directly changing the names of six biologics for which biosimilar applications remain in some phase of review.[47] **Table 8-3** illustrates the application of this proposed naming approach as well as the names for approved biologics since publication of this final guidance.[29-33,47-49]

TABLE 8-3. Proposed and Assigned Biological Names[29-33,47-49]

Brand name	Current Nonproprietary Name	Proposed Nonproprietary Name (i.e., proper name)
Neupogen	Filgrastim	Filgrastim-jcwp
Granix	Tbo-filgrastim	Filgrastim-vkzt
Epogen/Procrit	Epoetin alfa	Epoetin alfa-cgkn
Neulasta	Pegfilgrastim	Pegfilgrastim-lfjd
Remicade	Infliximab	Infliximab-hjmt
Zarxio	Filgrastim-sndz	Filgrastim-bflm
Inflectra	Inflixkmab-dyyb	N/A
Erelzi	Etanercept-szzs	N/A
Amjevita	Adalimumab-atto	N/A
Renflexis	Infliximab-abda	N/A
Cyltezo	Adalimumab-adbm	N/A
Mvasi	Bevacizumzb-awwb	N/A

N/A = not applicable.

Prior to the publication of this guidance, FDA approved its first biosimilar with a place-holder name, filgrastim-sndz.[47] As described in Table 8-3, this product has received a different proposed suffix that eliminates the abbreviation of the manufacturer.[47] Since the publication of this guidance's draft version, additional biosimilar agents have been approved including versions of infliximab, etanercept, adalimumab, and bevacizumab.[29-33,48,49] Those agents have received the proper names infliximab-dyyb, etanercept-szzs, adalimumab-atto, infliximab-abda, adalimumab-adbm, and bevacizumab-awwb.[29-33,48,49]

According to the FDA guidance document on naming, the integration of a suffix into the nonproprietary name is intended to prevent inadvertent substitution and promote pharmacovigilance.[45] Also, FDA has stated that the application of the naming convention to all biological products is intended to encourage routine use of designated suffixes in ordering, prescribing, dispensing, and recordkeeping practices, and to avoid inaccurate perceptions of the safety and effectiveness of biological products.[45]

While some organizations have supported the application of a unique suffix, others have questioned the utility of this decision and whether it achieves the desired goal of promoting pharmacovigilance.[37,44] The strategy of utilizing a suffix that is intentionally devoid of meaning would appear to make recollection more difficult and allow ordering of a product that is not desired, encourage the documentation of an incomplete name (without the suffix), and increase the likelihood of transcription of a suffix that does not exist.[50] In addition, it is unknown to what extent the electronic medical record, pharmacy information system, and drug information vendors will be able to incorporate this attribute into their databases and if their approach to this change in nomenclature will be the same.[50]

It is also noted that the FDA approach, while similar, is distinct from the WHO guidance in several circumstances. The WHO has adopted an approach of using a unique identifier called a *biologic qualifier* (BQ) of four random consonants in two 2-letter blocks separated by a 2-digit checksum.[46] The WHO scheme is intended to provide a uniform global means of identification of biologic drugs and avoid the proliferation of differing national schemes.[46] As FDA has chosen a different approach, there will be variation in the U.S. identification of biologics as compared to other nations that choose the BQ approach.

COLLECTING MEANINGFUL DATA

Although the biosimilar approval process is designed to support the introduction of highly similar products that possess no clinically meaningful differences in safety, purity, or potency, validation of the perspective is desirable. As previously discussed, existing pharmacovigilance methods, even of small molecule drugs, has revealed gaps and absences of needed data.[39,40] Therefore, FDA and other organizations are continuing to investigate additional approaches to obtain needed surveillance information. One recently announced approach is that of the Biologics and Biosimilars Collective Intelligence Consortium (BBCIC), a nonprofit, public service initiative.[51] BBCIC, although established by the Academy of Managed Care Pharmacy, is a separate entity with its own distinct budget and governing structure.[51] The BBCIC draws on large datasets of de-identified pharmacy and medical claims data to monitor the effectiveness and safety of novel biologics, their corresponding biosimilars, and other related products.[51] BBCIC utilizes the same scientific and analytical methods as FDA's Sentinel Initiative, a post-market surveillance network that has access to claims and other data for more than 190 million individuals.[51]

BBCIC is a collaboration of managed care organizations, integrated delivery systems, pharmacy benefit managers, research institutions, and pharmaceutical companies.[51] Participating pharmaceutical companies include AbbVie, Amgen, Boehringer-Ingelheim, Merck, Momenta, and Pfizer.[51] BBCIC is conducting a range of analyses, including population characterization, epidemiologic studies, and active observational sequential analysis of biologics and biosimilars.[51] Initial areas of research include product categories for which biosimilars are expected in the next few years including the tumor necrosis factor–alpha inhibitors and epoetin alfa.[51]

LOOK ALIKE AND SOUND ALIKE, BUT NOT TOO MUCH

The structure and implementation of the BPCI Act is to ensure that licensed biosimilars are thoroughly scrutinized so that the potential for adverse events, including immunogenicity, is the same as that of the originator branded product.[7] As a result, biosimilars are highly comparable to their reference counterparts.[7] However, all biologics, both biosimilars and branded agents, will be differentiated through their nonproprietary name, specifically their proper names.[45] How should pharmacists navigate this landscape of products that are neither identical nor totally different, especially in the context of supporting patient safety? Pharmacists must pre-emptively consider all elements of biologics to ensure appropriate differentiation when required for operational purposes without conflating these differences with any variations in clinical safety or efficacy.

Biosimilars will possess differing brand and nonproprietary names.[29-33] Therefore, the first consideration is how to distinguish these products throughout the myriad of clinical, operational, and financial information systems that manage data about prescription pharmaceuticals.[52,53] Will the agents be designated via their brand name, proper (i.e., nonproprietary) name, or both?[53] With the products already launched, we have seen issues where the biosimilar version is not available in all of these dosage forms manufactured for the brand.[54] How will this variation affect use, particularly when injection devices and pens become available for self-administered products?[31,32] Similarly, clinicians and patients have likely become familiar with the labeling and packaging of originator products. Biosimilar packaging might resemble the originator, or may differ significantly.[52] How will these differences be managed to prevent inadvertent confusion? These issues are all relevant when simply considering a comprehensive change from one product to the other. Pharmacies may have to maintain multiple related agents (originator and biosimilars) on formulary depending on payer coverage. As a result, the need to distinguish and differentiate products is even more critical.

Therapeutic interchange strategies can likely inform a lot of our efforts in this arena.[55] Health-system pharmacists are very much accustomed to establishing therapeutic interchange programs where molecularly distinct agents with differing dosage forms, names, dosage regimens, etc., are substituted for each other.[55] The key to success is ensuring that all clinicians and other stakeholders that will be managing some part of the medication process understand the relationship of the drugs for which substitution is taking place.[55] Education is critically important along with reinforcement via reminders, alerts, and other notifications.

Biosimilars are pharmaceuticals and just like their originator reference products, their use will result in adverse events. As a result, it is important to identify and document these occurrences. It is also important to view these events, both in terms of frequency and type, in the context of the information we should be currently capturing regarding the use and outcomes associated with branded biologics. The level of rigor associated with biosimilar review does not exempt us from effective pharmacovigilance strategies. Instead, biosimilars offer another opportunity for health-system pharmacists to improve the level of surveillance for all outcomes associated with pharmaceutical care.

KEY POINTS

- All medications, small molecule and biologic, originator and generic/biosimilar can cause adverse events. The risk of immunogenicity is greater with biologics, both originator and biosimilar, due to their size and complexity.

- Biosimilars in highly regulated markets, such as the United States and European Union, are rigorously evaluated to ensure there are no clinically meaningful differences in safety profiles.

- Adverse events will occur with biosimilars just as they do with biologics. Therefore, appropriate pharmacovigilance strategies are necessary to ensure safe and effective use.

CONCLUSION

The approach to biosimilar pharmacovigilance involves an expectation of due diligence. Given the rigorous standards required for biosimilar approval, we would not expect a higher degree of safety issues as compared to originator reference products. Nevertheless, the need for improved adverse event documentation and tracking for all medications should be a deliberate goal for pharmacists. In addition, the collection and analysis of biosimilar specific safety data will help foster a greater level of confidence in this new class of biologics. Pharmacists must ensure that appropriate mechanisms are in place to capture and review this information.

REFERENCES

1.   Weise M, Bielsky MC, De Smet K et al. Biosimilars: what clinicians should know. *Blood.* 2012; 120:5111-7.

2.   Praditpornsilpa K, Tiranathanagul K, Kupatawintu P et al. Biosimilar recombinant human erythropoietin induces the production of neutralizing antibodies. *Kidney Int.* 2011; 80:88-92.

3.   Bennett CL, Luminari S, Nissenson AR. Pure red-cell aplasia and epoetin therapy. *N Engl J Med.* 2004; 351:1403-8.

4.   Vermeer NS, Spierings I, Mantel-Teeuwisse AK et al. Traceability of biologicals: present challenges in pharmacovigilance. *Expert Opin Drug Saf.* 2015; 14:63-72.

5.   Purcell RT, Lockley RF. Immunologic responses to therapeutic biologic agents. *J Investig Allergol Clin Immunol.* 2008; 18:335-42.

6.   Kessler M, Goldsmith D, Schellekens H. Immunogenicity of biopharmaceuticals. *Nephol Dial Transplant* 2006; 21 Supply 5:v9-v12.

7.   Title VII: Improving access to innovative medical therapies. Subtitle A: Biologic Price Competition and Innovation provisions of the Patient Protection and Affordable Care Act (PPACA). www.fda.gov/downloads/Drugs/GuidanceComplianceRegulatoryInformation/ucm216146.pdf (accessed 1 Oct 2017).

8.   Food and Drug Administration. Guidance for industry. Scientific considerations in demonstrating biosimilarity to a reference product, April 2015. www.fda.gov/downloads/drugs/guidancecomplianceregulatoryinformation/guidances/ucm291128.pdf (accessed 1 Oct 2017).

9.   Food and Drug Administration. Guidance for industry, draft guidance. Labeling for biosimilar products. www.fda.gov/downloads/drugs/guidancecomplianceregulatoryinformation/guidances/ucm493439.pdf (accessed 1 Oct 2017).

10. Clarke JB. Mechanisms of adverse drug reactions to biologics. In: *Adverse Drug Reactions, Handbook of Experimental Pharmacology.* J. Uetrecht (ed.). Springer-Verlag Berlin Heidelberg 2010:452-74.

11. Baldo BA. Approved biologics used for therapy and their adverse effects. In: *Safety of Biologics Therapy.* Springer International Publishing Switzerland 2016:1-27.

12. Remicade (infliximab) package insert. Horsham, PA: Janssen Biotech, Inc; October 2015.

13. Humira (adalimumab) package insert. North Chicago, IL: AbbVie, Inc; April 2017.

14. Enbrel (etanercept) package insert. Thousand Oaks, CA; Immunex Corporation; November 2016.

15. Rituxan (rituximab) package insert. South San Francisco, CA; Genentech; April 2016.

16. Singh SK. Impact of product-related factors on immunogenicity of biotherapeutics. *J Pharm Sci.* 2011; 100:354-87.

17. Rosenberg AS, Verthelyi D, Cherney BW. Managing uncertainty: a perspective on risk pertaining to product quality attributes as they bear on immunogenicity of therapeutic proteins. *J Pharm Sci.* 2012; 101:3560-7.

18. Al-Sabbagh A, Olech E, McClellan JE, Kirchhoff CF. Development of biosimilars. *Semin Arthritis Rheum.* 2016; 45(5 Suppl):S11-8.

19. McKoy JM, Stonecash RE, Cournoyer D et al. Epoetin-associated pure red cell aplasia: past, present, and future considerations. *Transfusion.* 2008; 48:1754-62.

20. Casadevall N, Eckardt KU, Rossert J. Epoetin-induced autoimmune pure red cell aplasia. *J Am Soc Nephrol.* 2005; 16:S67-9.

21. Creutzfeldt-Jakob Disease fact sheet. National Institute of Neurological Disorders and Stroke. https://www.ninds.nih.gov/Disorders/Patient-Caregiver-Education/Fact-Sheets/Creutzfeldt-Jakob-Disease-Fact-Sheet. (accessed 1 Oct 2017).

22. Ebbers HC, Mantel-Teeuwisse AK, Moors EH et al. Today's challenges in pharmacovigilance: what can we learn from epoetins? *Drug Saf.* 2011; 34:372-87.

23. Covic A, Abraham I. State-of-the-art biosimilar erythropoietins in the management of renal anemia: lessons learned from Europe and implications for US nephrologists. *Int Urol Nephrol.* 2015; 47:1529-39.

24. Casadevall N, Thorpe R, Schellekens H. Biosimilars need comparative clinical data. *Kidney Int.* 2011; 80:553.

25. Wish JB. The approval process for biosimilar erythropoiesis-stimulating agents. *Clin J Am Soc Nephrol.* 2014; 9:1645-51.

26. Seidl A, Hainzl O, Richter M et al. Tungsten-induced denaturation and aggregation of epoetin alfa during primary packaging as a cause of immunogenicity. *Pharm Res.* 2012; 29:1454-67.

27. GABI Online. New administration route for epoetin alfa biosimilar Binocrit. www.gabionline.net/ Biosimilars/News/New-administration-route-for-epoetin-alfa-biosimilar-Binocrit (accessed 1 Oct 2017).

28. Strand B, Balsa A, Al-Saleh J et al. Immunogenicity of biologics in chronic inflammatory diseases: a systematic review. *BioDrugs.* 2017 June 13 [Epub ahead of print].

29. Zarxio (filgrastim-sndz) package insert. Princeton, NJ: Sandoz Inc; March 2015.

30. Inflectra (infliximab-dyyb) package insert. Yeonsu-gu, Incheon: Celltrion, Inc; April 2016.

31. Erelzi (etanercept-szzs) package insert. Princeton, NJ: Sandoz Inc; August 2016.

32. Amjevita (adalimumab-atto) package insert. Thousand Oaks, CA: Amgen; September 2016.

33. Renflexis (infliximab-abda) package insert. Yeonsu-gu, Incheon: Samsung Bioepsis: April 2017.

34. FDA briefing document. Oncologic Drugs Advisory Committee Meeting. May 25, 2017. BLA 125545. "Epoetin Hospira," a proposed biosimilar to Epogen/Procrit (epoetin alfa). www.fda.gov/ downloads/AdvisoryCommittees/CommitteesMeetingMaterials/Drugs/OncologicDrugsAdvisory-Committee/UCM559967.pdf (accessed 1 Oct 2017).

35. Quality considerations in demonstrating biosimilarity of a therapeutic protein product to a reference product. Guidance for industry. April 2015. www.fda.gov/downloads/drugs/guidancecompliance-regulatoryinformation/guidances/ucm291134.pdf (accessed 1 Oct 2017).

36. Boehm G, Yao L, Han L, Zheng Q. Development of the generic drug industry in the US after the Hatch-Waxman Act of 1984. *Acta Pharmaceutica Sinica B.* 2013; 3:297-311.

37. Hawana J. The contentious nonproprietary naming debate. www.law360.com/articles/682940/ the-contentious-biosimilar-nonproprietary-naming-debate (subscription) (accessed 1 Oct 2017).

38. Schiestl M, Stangler T, Torell C et al. Acceptable changes in quality attributes of glycosylated biop-harmaceuticals. *Nat Biotechnol.* 2011; 29:310-2.

39. Dal Pan GJ. Ongoing challenges in pharmacovigilance. *Drug Saf.* 2014; 37:1-8.

40. Gonzalez-Gonzalez C, Lopez-Gonzalez E, Herdeiro MT, Figueira A. Strategies to improve adverse drug reaction reporting: a critical and systematic review. *Drug Saf.* 2013; 36:317-28.

41. Grampp G, Bonafede M, Felix T et al. Active and passive surveillance of enoxaparin generics: a case study relevant to biosimilars. *Expert Opin Drug Saf.* 2015; 14:349-60.

42. Grampp G, Felix T. Pharmacovigilance considerations for biosimilars in the USA. *BioDrugs.* 2015; 29:309-21.

43. Biosimilars approved in Europe. GaBi online. www.gabionline.net/Biosimilars/General/Biosimi-lars-approved-in-Europe (accessed 1 Oct 2017).

44. Silverman E. Biosimilars: what's in a name? *BMJ.* 2014; 348:g272.

45. Food and Drug Administration. Guidance for industry. Nonproprietary naming of biological prod-ucts, draft guidance, August 2015. www.fda.gov/downloads/drugs/guidancecomplianceregulatory-information/guidances/ucm459987.pdf (accessed 1 Oct 2017).

46. Biological Qualifier, an INN Proposal. World Health Organization. www.who.int/medicines/ services/inn/WHO_INN_BQ_proposal_2015.pdf?ua=1 (accessed 1 Oct 2017).

47. Designation of official names and proper names for certain biological products. A proposed rule by the Food and Drug Administration on 08/28/2015. Federal Register. www.federalregister.gov/ documents/2015/08/28/2015-21382/designation-of-official-names-and-proper-names-for-cer-tain-biological-products (accessed 1 Oct 2017).

48. Cyltezo (adalimumab-abdm) package insert. Ridgefield, CT: Boehringer Ingelheim Pharmaceuticals, Inc; August, 2017.

49. Mvasi (bevacizumab-awwb) package insert. Thousand Oaks, CA: Amgen; September, 2017.

50. Siegel JF, Royzman I. Stakeholders say biosimilars names should be meaningful and memorable. www.biologicsblog.com/blog/stakeholders-say-biosimilars-names-should-be-meaningful-and-memorable/ (accessed 1 Oct 2017).

51. About the BBCIC. Biologics & Biosimilars Collective Intelligence Consortium. www.bbcic.org/ (accessed 1 Oct 2017).

52. Griffith N, McBride A, Stevenson JG, Green L. Formulary selection criteria for biosimilars: considerations for US health-system pharmacists. *Hosp Pharm*. 2014; 49:813-25.

53. Stevenson JG, Popovian R, Jacobs I et al. Biosimilars: practical considerations for pharmacists. *Ann Pharmacother*. 2017; 51:590-602.

54. Barlas S. Early biosimilars face hurdles to acceptance; the FDA has approved few, so lack of competition is keeping prices high. *PT*. 2016; 41:362-5.

55. Tyler LS, Cole SW, May JR et al. ASHP guidelines on the pharmacy and therapeutics committee and the formulary system. *Am J Health Syst Pharm*. 2008; 65:1272-83.

CHAPTER 9

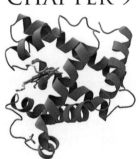

THE PATENT DANCE AND THE EXCLUSIVITY SHUFFLE

As pharmacists, our primary concern regarding the Biologics Price Competition and Innovation (BPCI) Act is the processes by which biosimilars are determined to be highly similar to their originator counterparts and the information that will govern their prescribing, use, and monitoring. Still, a fully-vetted biosimilar will make no contribution to the goal of lowering the costs of biologic therapy if its manufacturer cannot legally market the product. This chapter introduces the critical legal considerations that along with regulatory approval define the biosimilar market entry timeline so preparatory actions for formulary addition can be planned and implemented in the most efficient and timely manner. As with other elements of this discussion, to understand this new model, we should first start with what has previously existed.

EXCLUSIVITY AND PATENT PROTECTION

The generic drug era began in 1984 with the enactment of the Drug Price Competition and Patent Term Restoration Act, more commonly known as the *Hatch-Waxman Amendments*.[1,2] Most clinicians have likely fixated on this statute's components involving drug price competition. However, while Hatch-Waxman enabled a more efficient approach to generic drug approval, it also provided originator manufacturers the opportunity to recover some of the patent protection that otherwise would be lost in the investigational drug development process.[1,2]

It is important to understand that protection of branded pharmaceuticals from competition comes in two forms from two sources: exclusivity from the Food and Drug Administration (FDA) and patent protection from the U.S. Patent and Trademark Office (PTO).[3] These elements are similar yet different. Surprise! Within the context of pharmaceutical research, patent protection is usually sought first.[4] Early in the development of a new molecular entity, a manufacturer or drug developer will request a patent from PTO to protect the novelty of their product.[4] Patents can be requested throughout the life cycle of a drug's development.[3] If approved, the recipient receives protection for the patented element for 20 years from the date of filing.[3] A patent protects an innovator against other parties using their invention to develop a competing product.[4]

Separate from this process, as the new molecular entity proceeds through additional development, a manufacturer will ultimately file an investigational new drug (IND) application, which enables the progression of drug evaluation through the steps of Phase I, II, and III clinical trials.[3] For molecules that complete these steps successfully, the manufacturer will ultimately file and ideally receive approval of a new drug application (NDA). Once approved, the manufacturer receives a period of five years of exclusivity from the date of approval if the pharmaceutical is a new chemical entity.[3,4] Exclusivity periods can vary by product type as shown in **Table 9-1**.[4]

During this exclusivity period, other manufacturers are prohibited from submitting and receiving approval for a competing generic product.[4]

Although patent protection and marketing exclusivity are separate provisions, they both protect originator manufacturers from competition.[3] Also, while patent protection is technically for a longer duration, the benefit to the patent holder can still be greatly diminished given the time required to move a product from initial development through final NDA approval, on average 10 years.[5] This investment in time can significantly shorten the duration of functional

TABLE 9-1. Marketing Exclusivity for New Drug Applications[4]

Type of Exclusivity	Duration	Comments
New chemical entity (NCE)	5 years	■ Granted to a drug that contains no active moiety that has been approved by FDA under section 505(b) ■ Runs from time of NDA approval ■ Bars FDA from accepting for review any ANDA or 505(b)(2) application for a drug containing the same active moiety for: ● Five years if an ANDA or 505(b)(2) does not contain a paragraph IV certification to a listed patent ■ Four years if an ANDA or 505(b)(2) is submitted containing a paragraph IV certification to a listed patent
Orphan drug exclusivity (ODE)	7 years	■ Granted to drugs designated and approved to treat diseases or conditions affecting fewer than 200,000 in the United States (or more than 200,000 and no hope of recovering costs) ■ Runs from time of approval of NDA or BLA ■ Bars FDA from approving any other application [ANDA, 505(b)(2) or full NDA or BLA] for the same drug for the same orphan disease or condition
"Other" exclusivity	3 years	■ Granted to drug when application or supplement contains reports of new clinical investigations (not bioavailability studies conducted or sponsored by application and essential for approval) ■ Runs from time of NDA approval ■ Bars FDA from approving, for a 3-year period, any ANDA or 505(b)(2)
Pediatric exclusivity (PED)	6 months added to existing patents/ exclusivity	■ Grants an additional 6 months of market protection at the end of the listed patents and/or exclusivity for sponsor's drug products containing the active moiety, when the sponsor has conducted and submitted pediatric studies on the active moiety in response to a Written Request from FDA ■ Pediatric exclusivity takes on characteristics of 5-year, 3-year, or orphan exclusivity when it attaches to those protections.

ANDA = abbreviated new drug application; BLA = biologics license application; FDA = Food and drug Administration; NDA = new drug application.

patent protection. However, Hatch-Waxman authorized a process by which manufacturers could recoup some of that lost time.[1] Following NDA approval, a manufacturer can request drug patent term restoration.[1] If granted by PTO, manufacturers can have up to 5 years of patent protection restored provided the total time of exclusivity following product approval does not exceed 14 years.[2]

BIOSIMILAR PATENTS AND EXCLUSIVITY

A New Timeline

In addition to establishing the process for follow-on product approval, the BPCI Act also set the parameters for biosimilar exclusivity.[6] The debate involving this aspect of the legislation was quite controversial.[7] Previously (as described in Chapter 1), recombinant biologic manufacturers had basically enjoyed indefinite market exclusivity as no mechanism for approval of competing products existed. With the implementation of the BPCI Act, that insulation against competition was limited to a defined period of time.[6] Exclusivity durations of anywhere from 7 years to 14 years were proposed, with the compromise of 12 years ultimately included in the final version of the legislation signed into law.[6,7] FDA cannot approve a biosimilar earlier than 12 years from the initial date of approval of the originator reference product.[6] In addition, the BPCI Act also limits FDA from accepting a biosimilar application until four years after the initial approval of the reference originator biologic.[5] Given the increasing costs of all pharmaceuticals including biologics, there have been continued calls to lower this period of exclusivity to less than 12 years, although no such change thus far has been enacted.[7] Even though the general timeframe for biologic exclusivity appears to have been settled, pharmacists should not expect biosimilars to arrive exactly 12 years from the date of the originator's approval. As with generics, numerous factors influence when a competing product can enter the market. Many other aspects regarding patent infringement will also impact the timing of biosimilar launch. The BPCI Act includes a mechanism to navigate the patent infringement landscape.[6] This provision along with an intention to market notification requirement have both been the subject of numerous lawsuits culminating with a U.S. Supreme Court decision.[6,8] We will examine these issues and their impact on the timing of biosimilar launches in the next section.

What Type of Patent?

As stated earlier, patent protection through PTO tends to last longer than exclusivity associated with FDA product approval.[4] Although the duration of exclusivity for biosimilars is 12 years, the influence of patent protection will still be very substantial and could remain the rate-limiting step to biosimilar entry even after this deadline.[8] As described in previous chapters, biologics are built on the innovation of recombinant technology.[9] These innovations are highly proprietary and patent protected.[9] Even at the point in time the exclusivity period expires for the originator biologic molecule, the technology used to manufacture that product could remain confidential.[9] As a result, biosimilar sponsors must use different manufacturing processes to produce their highly similar versions of the same biologic molecule.[9] However, while biosimilar manufacturers would be expected to attempt to avoid patent infringement, there will undoubtedly be situations where potential conflicts are called into question. The BPCI Act included a process for patent litigation, commonly described as the *patent dance*.[6,10]

The Patent Dance, World War II, and the Quest for Clarity

In October 1939, Winston Churchill commented on the actions of Russia as "a riddle wrapped in a mystery inside an enigma."[11] Recently, a U.S. Court of Appeals judge referenced this quote in his assessment of the biosimilar *patent dance*, highlighting the continued complexity and varying interpretation of different aspects of this process.[11] The controversy regarding the patent dance begins with the very start of the process, the "apparent" requirement to disclose confidential information.[6] According to the BPCI Act, within 20 days of FDA accepting a 351(k) filing, the biosimilar applicant "shall provide to the reference product sponsor a copy of the application... and other information that describes the process or processes used to manufacture" the biosimilar.[6,12] From this point, the biosimilar and originator company exchange lists in a process (see **Table 9-2**) to try and agree on the patents that will be the subject of initial litigation.[6] Each of these steps has a defined time limit for response. Given that the statute uses the word "shall" in defining the biosimilar applicant's responsibility, it would seem that compliance with this exchange is non-negotiable.[6,12] Nevertheless, some biosimilar applicants have chosen to adopt an optional approach due to a reluctance to disclose the confidential elements of their application and proprietary manufacturing processes.[8,13] The initial case in which this consideration was litigated involved a dispute between Amgen versus Sandoz.[11] Through both a district and federal circuit court trial, the patent dance was determined to be optional with biosimilar applicants having the discretion to refrain from complying with this provision and instead facing an immediate infringement action.[13] Biosimilar manufacturers have chosen differing strategies regarding the exchange of information ranging from total refusal to engage, partial exchange of data, or a more complete engagement and exchange of information.[8]

	TABLE 9-2. The Biosimilar Patent Litigation Process (i.e., The Patent Dance)[12]
1.	Within 20 days of 351(k) application acceptance by the FDA, the biosimilar applicant "shall provide" a copy of the application to the originator reference product sponsor along with other information that describes the manufacturing processes of the biosimilar.
2.	Within 60 days of receiving the application and the manufacturing information, the originator reference sponsor provides to the biosimilar applicant a list of patents where a claim of patent infringement could reasonably be asserted; and identifies patents on the list the originator would be willing to license to the biosimilar applicant.
3.	Within 60 days of receiving the list from the originator reference product sponsor, the biosimilar applicant provides on a "claim by claim basis" why each patent identified "is invalid, unenforceable, or will not be infringed" by the marketed biosimilar, or a statement that the biosimilar will not be marketed before the date that "such patent expires."
4.	Within 60 days of receiving the response from the biosimilar applicant, the originator reference product sponsor provides a response on a "claim by claim" basis as to why the patents identified will be infringed by the marketing of the biosimilar.
5.	After receipt of response, both parties have 15 days to negotiate which identified patents will be the subject of patent infringement negotiation. If both parties agree, the originator reference sponsor has 30 days to bring an action for patent infringement. If both sides do not agree, within 5 days, the biosimilar applicant and the originator applicant exchange individual lists of the patents each feels should be litigated. The originator reference sponsor then has 30 days to bring an action for patent infringement.

To Notify or Not to Notify, and If So When

The patent dance represents one key component of biosimilar litigation. Another element that has been similarly controversial is the requirement for the biosimilar sponsor to notify the originator reference product manufacturer of its intent to market its product.[6,8,12] The BPCI Act includes a requirement that a biosimilar sponsor provide 180 days advanced notice to the originator reference product manufacturer of their intent to market the competing product. This expectation ensures that originator suppliers are cognizant of competing products under development and provides them the opportunity to request that marketing of the biosimilar be stopped until patent infringement issues are resolved.[6] In this case, the controversy has focused not on whether this consideration is mandatory or optional, but at what point in time notification can be provided.[8,12] As with many aspects of the BPCI Act, the controversy has centered on the language used in the statute, specifically the expectation that the notice must occur "not later than 180 days before the date of the first commercial marketing of the biological product licensed under" the 351(k) biologics application pathway.[6] In other words, can the notification be provided prior to final product approval so that the date of final licensing and initial marketing coincide, or must biosimilar manufacturers wait and provide notification after approval? Requiring final licensing prior to notification extends the effective exclusivity of the originator manufacturer. Allowing notification to occur prior to final approval would favor biosimilar applicants in expediting the launch of their products. One argument against post-approval notification is the fact that the BPCI Act set the exclusivity period for originator biologics at 12 years.[14] By limiting the 180-day notification to post-approval products, the duration of exclusivity could be construed as 12.5 years.[14] Whereas the lower courts concluded in the patent dance that the choice of the word "shall" should be interpreted as optional, they conversely stated that the word "licensed" means notification can only occur after formal approval, thus delaying the launch of approved biosimilars like filgrastim-sndz and infliximab-dyyb to recognize the 180-day notification requirement.[15,16]

THE SUPREME COURT'S ANSWER

After numerous hearings and various rulings in multiple lower courts, the Supreme Court heard these two issues in the case of *Sandoz Inc v Amgen Inc* and, on June 12, 2017, rendered its decision, which appears initially at least to favor biosimilar applicants.[17] First, the Supreme Court ruled that the patent dance is in fact optional.[17] According to the Court's unanimous decision, the BPCI Act, which defines the federal law, does not give originator biologic manufacturers the right to seek an injunction for failure to comply with the requirements of the patent dance.[17] The justices did say that it is possible that some state laws, for example, California in the Amgen versus Sandoz case, might grant that authority.[17] The Supreme Court has sent back this aspect of the decision to the Federal Circuit Court to make this determination.[17] Second, the Court ruled that the 180-day notification can be given prior to final approval of the biosimilar in question, eliminating the additional six months of exclusivity that biosimilar products previously had to endure.[17] It also accelerated the date of launch for biosimilars like infliximab-abda, that have already been approved and for which relevant patents that could present infringement concerns have likely expired.[18]

The 180-day notification requirement appears to have been resolved. Biosimilar sponsors can provide this notice prior to final approval and avoid any additional delays for their products after FDA grants licensing. The patent dance issue has been defined from a federal standpoint, although it is possible state laws might make this process mandatory.[17] However, no time frame yet exists as to when a further determination might be made.

The Inter Partes Review Alternative

Although the patent dance has been determined to remain an optional consideration, patent litigation will remain a very visible component of biosimilar development. For example, even for companies that have chosen to comply fully with the patent exchange, the patent dance does not begin until FDA has formally accepted a biosimilar application for review.[6,12] From that point, the time required to navigate the patent dance, provided all the proposed time limits are met, would be an estimated 230 days.[6,12] Also, the actual work of litigating a patent infringement claim can easily take two years to complete.[19] In a district court, the patent holder enjoys a statutory presumption of validity. A petitioner has to prove that a patent claim is invalid by clear and convincing evidence.[20] Furthermore, a district court judge hearing a case may or may not have patent litigation experience and/or a technical background.[20] Given these challenges, biosimilar applicants have evaluated the opportunity of using the inter partes review (IPR) process as an alternative to these challenges.[21]

The *IPR process*, introduced in 2012 as part of the America Invents Act (AIA), is a procedure to challenge the validity of patent claims.[21] An IPR is a trial conducted by the Patent Trial and Appeal Board (PTAB) at PTO to review the patentability of one or more claims where the petitioner has demonstrated that there is a reasonable likelihood that they would prevail.[19,21] An IPR addresses many of the issues associated with district court trials.[20] For example, there is no presumption of validity in a PTAB proceedings, which represents a significantly reduced burden of proof.[19,20] The time required to conduct an IPR is shorter.[19,20] By statute, an IPR must be completed within one year of institution, although an extension of up to six months may be allowed if justified.[19,20] Administrative patent judges with significant patent experience, who often possess technical backgrounds, decide the IPRs.[19,20] The interest in this alternative pathway to invalidate patents and shorten the period of exclusivity of originator products is seen by the number of IPRs that have been requested and those that are pending.[22] At the time of writing, pending IPRs existed for adalimumab, rituximab, and trastuzumab.[22] While this avenue offers potential efficiencies to petitioners, it is not guaranteed to remove all patents that could prevent the introduction of biosimilar competition. This fact was recently illustrated when PTAB declined to institute an IPR on a patent for AbbVie's Humira (adalimumab) that Coherus had requested.[22] This decision could help delay biosimilar competition for this molecule until beyond 2022.[23]

WILL THE IPR PROCESS REMAIN?

The IPR process has been successful in helping to invalidate certain patents and open the door to earlier competition for biosimilar products.[24] This success combined with the Supreme Court's ruling regarding the patent dance, favor biosimilar developers.[17,24] However, the Supreme Court has agreed to hear a case that will determine if the IPR process is constitutional and if it will remain as an avenue for biosimilar manufacturers to remove patents that present barriers to competition.[25] The primary issue for this concern is whether the IPR process violates the Seventh Amendment to the Constitution by eliminating the right to a trial jury.[25] Even if the IPR process remains, originator manufacturers continue to take additional innovative approaches to mitigate their risks of exclusivity loss due to court proceedings. Allergen recently made headlines in its efforts to insulate its product Restasis (cyclosporine ophthalmic solution) from IPR action by transferring ownership of key patents to a Native American tribe, a sovereign entity presumably immune to patent challenges at the PTAB.[26]

Finally, AbbVie and Amgen recently announced an agreement concerning the originator biologic Humira (adalimumab). Under this agreement, Amgen would cease its patent litigation activities in exchange for the right to launch its biosimilar of Humira, Amjevita (adalimumab-atto) on January 31, 2023.[27] Whether it is patent litigation, IPR proceedings, or settlements to discontinue various legal actions, many factors beyond FDA approval determine when a manufacturer has the right to launch a biosimilar product into the U.S. market.

WHY SHOULD A PHARMACIST CARE ABOUT PATENT LAW?

The essential opportunity afforded by biosimilars is lower prices, which obviously affects the budgeting process. Given the complexity and newness of the biosimilar concept, a greater investment in formulary review and education will be required.[28] Therefore, pharmacists must also allocate adequate resources to support the formulary and financial analysis needed for biosimilar review. Due to this investment of time, attention, and educational support, it is critical pharmacists understand all of the factors that will determine when a biosimilar actually reaches the market. If a product is approved, but delayed in its launch, a pharmacy executive cannot include potential financial savings in their budget cycle forecast. Also, given the limited resources available in all healthcare institutions, pharmacist leaders must know when clinical formulary support will be required. If an approved biosimilar will not launch for several years, application of resources to other activities might present a more efficient use of personnel and expertise. Finally, patent limitations may have an impact beyond just molecule availability and actually affect patient acceptance of a biosimilar.[29]

THE PATIENT CARE EXPERIENCE OF PATENT LAW

There are many elements of a medication that can be patented including the molecule itself, its development and manufacturing processes, the way in which it is used, and even the formulation used to deliver the product.[29] This fact is particularly important with biologic medications, especially those that are self-administered. As biologic drugs must be delivered parenterally, they are provided in various injectable formulations including syringes. However, these formulations can be patent protected, necessitating the development of alternative methods for administration.[29] As a result, self-administered biosimilars will not be in identical delivery devices as the originators.[28] These products will be different and will necessitate substantial educational efforts to ensure complete and comprehensive understanding of patients and their caregivers.[28] While currently not considered a biosimilar, the introduction of a follow-on version of somatropin (Omnitrope; Sandoz) was limited because the initial formulation was a lyophilized vial, which required substantial manipulation.[30] Sandoz has since launched a prefilled syringe.[30] Again, these issues will become more evident as biosimilars for self-administered biologics like adalimumab and etanercept are finally launched in the market.[31,32]

THE CHANGING CLINICAL PRACTICE LANDSCAPE

The introduction of biosimilars will necessitate a substantial degree of education and support to gain the acceptance of these agents as comparable alternatives to the originator reference products that define the standard of care for many disease states. However, the definition of the standard of care is not static as the pharmaceutical industry continues to innovate and introduce new molecules that not only offer treatment alternatives against which biosimilars must compete, but also renew the originators' exclusivity for their product pipelines. Frequently, these types of developments are characterized as biobetters.[33]

Currently, there is no statutory definition of a biobetter.[33] However, proposed definitions for these second- or next-generation products include biologicals that have been structurally and/ or functionally altered to achieve an improved or different clinical performance.[34] Even within the originator biopharmaceutical development process, examples of innovation and continued advancement have been seen within the granulocyte colony stimulating factor and erythropoietin classes.[35] The introduction of pegfilgrastim and darbepoetin allowed for extended dosing, improving clinician and patient convenience.[35] It should also be noted that enhancements could include strategies beyond just a molecular modification, but also involve a change in dosage form and/or route of administration.[36,37] **Table 9-3** lists some recently approved and anticipated enhanced biologics and/or presentations of existing originator molecule.[35-44]

Due to this continuing level of innovation, a biosimilar will be unlikely to capture the totality of the originator's potential use as prescribing habits will already be migrating to other origina-

TABLE 9-3. New Products/Next Generation Enhancements for Commonly Used Biologics[35-44]	
Existing Agent	**Modification**
Neulasta (pegfilgrastim)	■ Pegfilgrastim auto injector (Neulasta OnPro)*
Rituxan (rituximab) intravenous injection	■ Rituximab subcutaneous*
	■ Obinutuzumab*
Herceptin (trastuzumab)	■ Trastuzumab 150 mg vial*
	■ Pertuzumab*
	■ Ado-trastuzumab emtansine*
Remicade (infliximab)	■ Secukinumab*
Humira (adalimumab)	■ Ustekinumab*
Enbrel (etancercept)	■ Vedolizumab*
	■ Sarilumab*
	■ Guselkumab (IL-23 inhibitor for plaque psoriasis)*
	■ Upadacitinib (Janus kinase-1 inhibitor for rheumatoid arthritis)
	■ Risankizumab (IL-23 inhibitor for psoriasis)
	■ Tildrakinzumab (IL-23 inhibitor for psoriasis)*

*Approved.

tors. Pharmacists must monitor this impact as they attempt to establish accurate estimates of the potential value biosimilar use could bring to their organizations. Similarly, pharmacists must evaluate novel biologics or new formulations of existing biologics to assess the true value these products bring to the market as compared to the value afforded by biosimilars.

Key Points

■ Beyond approval considerations, many legal issues affect the timing for the launch of biosimilars and even the formulations in which biosimilars can be marketed.

■ Pharmacists must remain vigilant of court rulings that could either remove or reinforce barriers to biosimilar market entry.

■ Such information helps pharmacists in determining the timeline for resource support of biosimilar launch and assessing the extent of financial savings that could be realized.

Conclusion

A biosimilar cannot be launched prior to it receiving final approval from FDA. However, another critical element that will govern the timing of launch, particularly during this initial phase of biosimilar development, will be the resolution of legal issues surrounding these products. Biologics are the result of substantial technological innovation, which benefits patient populations and contributes to the use of originator medications. However, the same innovation and proprietary information that allow for these products also present numerous hurdles for the introduction of competition. In addition, the interpretations of various aspects of the review process remain unsettled. The recent final ruling regarding the patent dance and the timing of the 180-day notification requirement have helped clarify the legal landscape. Nevertheless, litigation will remain an important influence on the timing of biosimilar launches, which pharmacists should monitor closely for changes that will accelerate or delay the introduction of competing products.

REFERENCES

1. Asclone FJ, Kirking DM, Gaither CA, Welage LS. Historical overview of generic medication policy. *J Am Pharm Assoc*. 2001; 41:567-77.
2. Boehm G, Yao Lixin, Han Liang, Zheng Q. Development of the generic drug industry in the US after the Hatch-Waxman Act of 1984. *Acta Pharmaceutica Sinica B*. 2013; 3:297-311.
3. Frequently asked questions on patents and exclusivity. Food and Drug Administration. www.fda.gov/Drugs/DevelopmentApprovalProcess/ucm079031.htm (accessed 2 Oct 2017).
4. Patents and Exclusivity. FDA/CDER SBIA Chronicles, May 19, 2015. www.fda.gov/downloads/drugs/developmentapprovalprocess/smallbusinessassistance/ucm447307.pdf (accessed 2 Oct 2017).
5. Biopharmaceutical Research & Development: The Process behind New Markets. PhRMA. http://phrma-docs.phrma.org/sites/default/files/pdf/rd_brochure_022307.pdf (accessed Oct. 2, 2017).

6. Title VII: Improving access to innovative medical therapies. Subtitle A: Biologic Price Competition and Innovation provisions of the Patient Protection and Affordable Care Act (PPACA). www.fda.gov/downloads/Drugs/GuidanceComplianceRegulatoryInformation/ucm216146.pdf (accessed 2 Oct 2017).

7. Carver KH, Elikan J, Lietzan E. An unofficial legislative history of the Biologics Price Competition and Innovation Act of 2009. *Food Drug Law J.* 2010; 65:670-818.

8. BPCIA Litigation Summary Chart. Big Molecule Watch. www.bigmoleculewatch.com/bpcia-litigation-summary-chart/ (accessed 2 Oct 2017).

9. Mellstedt H, Niederwieser D, Ludwig H. The challenge of biosimilars. *Ann Oncol.* 2008; 19:411-9.

10. Malkin BJ. Biosimilars patent litigation in the EU and the US: a comparative strategic overview. *GaBI J.* 2015; 4:113-7. http://gabi-journal.net/biosimilars-patent-litigation-in-the-eu-and-the-us-a-comparative-strategic-overview.html (accessed 2 Oct 2017).

11. Amgen Inc., Amgen Manufacturing Limited vs. Sandoz Inc., 2015–1499. http://www.cafc.uscourts.gov/sites/default/files/s15-1499.pdf (accessed 2 Oct 2017).

12. Sensabaugh SM. Requirements for biosimilars and interchangeable biological drugs in the United States—in plain language. *Drug Inf J.* 2011; 45:155-62.

13. BPCIA litigation roundup (Fall 2016). www.bigmoleculewatch.com/2016/11/23/bpcia-litigation-roundup-fall-2016/ (accessed 2 Oct 2017).

14. Brennan Z. GPhA's Biosimilars Council: BPCIA providers 12 years exclusivity, not 12.5. www.raps.org/Regulatory-Focus/News/2016/01/07/23855/GPhA%E2%80%99s-Biosimilars-Council-BPCIA-Provides-12-Years-Exclusivity-Not-125/ (accessed 2 Oct 2017).

15. Sandoz launches Zarxio (filgrastim-sndz), the first biosimilar in the United States. Press release. www.novartis.com/news/media-releases/sandoz-launches-zarxiotm-filgrastim-sndz-first-biosimilar-united-states (accessed 2 Oct 2017).

16. Bulik BS. For Inflectra launch, Pfizer uses 'hybrid model' to home in on HCPs. www.fiercepharma.com/marketing/pfizer-s-inflectra-biosimilar-launch-marks-new-go-to-market-strategy (accessed 2 Oct 2017).

17. Brennan Z. US Supreme Court: no six-month wait for biosimilars after FDA approval. www.raps.org/Regulatory-Focus/News/2017/06/12/27881/US-Supreme-Court-No-Six-Month-Wait-for-Biosimilars-After-FDA-Approval/ (accessed 2 Oct 2017)

18. Sagonowsky E. Targeting a $5B brand, Samsung and Merck launch Remicade biosim at 35% discount. http://www.fiercepharma.com/pharma/samsung-merck-launch-remicade-biosim-at-35-discount (accessed 2 Oct 2017).

19. Flibbert MJ, Queler MD. 5 distinctions between IPRs and district court patent litigation. www.finnegan.com/resources/articles/articlesdetail.aspx?news=64c22ef3-9abe-4637-a445-c75c56892eb1 (accessed 2 Oct 2017).

20. Inter Partes Review (IPR): an alternative pathway for biosimilars. IP Reports, March 2015. www.bakerbotts.com/ideas/publications/2015/03/ptab-trials-report2 (accessed 2 Oct 2017).

21. Inter Partes Review. Fish & Richardson. http://fishpostgrant.com/inter-partes-review/ (accessed 2 Oct 2017).

22. Inter Partes Review. Big Molecule Watch. www.bigmoleculewatch.com/iprs/ (accessed 2 Oct 2017).

23. Helfand C. AbbVie's Humira gets an IP boost as PTO strikes down Coherus challenge. www.fiercepharma.com/pharma/abbvie-s-humira-gets-ip-boost-as-pto-strikes-down-coherus-challenge (accessed 2 Oct 2017).

24. Pagliarulo N. Coherus wins Humira patent ruling, chipping away at AbbVie's defenses. www.biopharmadive.com/news/coherus-humira-patent-abbvie-ipr-biosimilar/442950/ (accessed 2 Oct 2017).

25. Sandburg B. PTAB tosses two more Humira patents; will Supreme Court Eliminate IPR Proceeding? *The Pink Sheet,* June 14, 2017.

26. Sagonowsky E. Mylan blasts Allergan's "desperate" tribal licensing deal on Restasis. www.fiercepharma.com/legal/mylan-blasts-allergan-s-desperate-tribal-licensing-deal-restasis (accessed 2 Oct 2017).

27. Sandburg B. Humira biosimilar settlement could be model for other disputes. *The Pink Sheet*, September 28, 2017.

28. Griffith N, McBride A, Stevenson JG, Green L. Formulary selection criteria for biosimilars: considerations for US Health-System Pharmacists. *Hosp Pharm*. 2014; 49:813-25.

29. Pollack A. Makers of Humira and Enbrel using new drug patents to delay generic versions. *The New York Times*, July 15, 2016. www.nytimes.com/2016/07/16/business/makers-of-humira-and-enbrel-using-new-drug-patents-to-delay-generic-versions.html?_r=0 (accessed 2 Oct 2017).

30. Fuhr U, Tuculanu D, Berghout A, et al. Bioequivalence between novel ready-to-use liquid formulations of the recombinant human GH Omnitrope and the original lyophilized formulations for reconsition of Omnitrope and Genotropin. *Eur J Endocrinol*. 2010; 162:1051-8. www.eje-online.org/content/162/6/1051.full.pdf (accessed 2 Oct 2017).

31. Erelzi (etanercept-szzs) package insert. Princeton, NJ: Sandoz Inc; August 2016.

32. Amjevita (adalimumab-atto) package insert. Thousand Oaks, CA: Amgen; September 2016.

33. Anour R. Biosimilars versus 'biobetters': a regulator's perspective. *GaBI J*. 2014; 3:166-7. http://gabi-journal.net/biosimilars-versus-biobetters-a-regulators-perspective.html (accessed 2 Oct 2017).

34. Weise M, Bielsky MC, De Smet K et al. Biosimilars—why terminology matters. *Nat Biotechnol*. 2011; 29:690-3.

35. Strohl WR. Fusion proteins for half-life extension of biologics as a strategy to make biobetters. *BioDrugs*. 2015; 29:215-39.

36. Saxena V. Amgen launches delivery device for automatic administration of its blockbuster Neulasta. www.fiercepharma.com/r-d/amgen-launches-delivery-device-for-automatic-administration-of-its-blockbuster-neulasta (accessed 2 Oct 2017).

37. FDA accepts Genentech's biologics license application for subcutaneous formulation of rituximab. Halozyme press release. www.halozyme.com/investors/news-releases/news-release-details/2016/FDA-Accepts-Genentechs-Biologics-License-Application-For-Subcutaneous-Formulation-Of-Rituximab/default.aspx (accessed Oct. 2, 2017).

38. Reichert JM. Antibodies to watch in 2017. *mAbs* 2017; 9:167-81.

39. Helfand C. Gazyva: Rituxan follow-up joins the next generation of Roche cancer blockbusters. www.fiercebiotech.com/special-report/gazyva-rituxan-follow-up-joins-next-generation-of-roche-cancer-blockbusters (accessed Oct. 2, 2017).

40. Blackstone EA, Joseph PF. The economics of biosimilars. *Am Health Drug Benefits*. 2013; 6:469-78.

41. AbbVie press release. AbbVie's upadacitinib (ABT-494) meets all primary and ranked secondary endpoints in phase 3 study in rheumatoid arthritis. www.prnewswire.com/news-releases/abbvies-upadacitinib-abt-494-meets-all-primary-and-ranked-secondary-endpoints-in-phase-3-study-in-rheumatoid-arthritis-300470191.html (accessed 2 Oct. 2017).

42. Williams S. This looks to be Johnson & Johnson's next blockbuster drug. www.fool.com/investing/2016/10/05/this-looks-to-be-johnson-johnsons-next-blockbuster.aspx (accessed 2 Oct 2017).

43. Drugs@FDA: FDA Approved Drug Products database. www.accessdata.fda.gov/scripts/cder/daf/index.cfm (accessed 2 Oct 2017).

44. Herceptin (trastuzumab) package insert. South San Francisco, CA: Genentech, Inc; April 2017.

CHAPTER 10

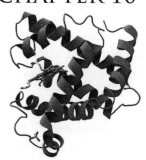

DEFINING BIOSIMILAR VALUE AND OTHER SEEMINGLY IMPOSSIBLE TASKS

The intrinsic purpose of biosimilars is to introduce direct competition for branded biologics thus lowering the cost for critical pharmaceuticals used in healthcare.[1] As has been established over decades of experience with generic medications, the availability of competitors following branded product loss of exclusivity helps decrease treatment expense.[2] The use of an abbreviated approval process for generics diminishes a manufacturer's financial investment allowing sale at a reduced acquisition price.[3] Although the biosimilar approval process is more rigorous than that of generics, the targeted and focused approach enables lower development costs, thus allowing for the marketing of a highly similar molecule at a price threshold lower than that of its originator comparator.[1,3] Unfortunately, the exact degree to which prices will be lower remains unknown given the formative state of the U.S. biosimilars market.[4] In addition, while all participants in healthcare desperately want to control biologic drug expenditures, the way they desire financial relief varies depending on where they reside within our ever more complicated pharmaceutical supply chain.[2,4] Among all of the complexities related to biosimilars, accurately predicting their value may ultimately prove to be the most challenging endeavor. We must appreciate the competing forces that are currently vying for biosimilar savings as pharmacy inherits the responsibility of translating these variables into a coherent financial model.

WHAT ESTIMATES OF SAVINGS CURRENTLY EXIST?

Within the continual conversation regarding the high prices of pharmaceuticals, a frequent topic of discussion is the cost of medication development and manufacturing. The most frequently cited estimate places the figure of developing a novel pharmaceutical, small molecule or biologic, at $2.6 billion.[5] In contrast, the estimated expense for creating a competing generic molecule is possibly as low as $1 million to $4 million with only two to three years of development time required.[3] Although the biosimilar pathway is intended to be more tailored, it will still require a greater level of manufacturing capability, analytical characterization work, and clinical support than generic approvals.[2] The predicted development costs range from $100 million to $250 million with a development window of seven to eight years.[3] As a result, while less expensive than novel drug development, the investment cost is more substantial than a generic program, which limits the degree of price lowering.[4] This higher threshold in terms of both manufacturing expertise and financial commitment will likely limit the number of market entrants able to exert downward influence on pricing.[3]

Given these considerations, rather than expecting the discounts of up to 80% that are sometimes seen with generics, the pricing concessions with biosimilars have been projected to range between 15% and 30%.[6] That estimate has thus far been validated with initially marketed biosimilars. Filgrastim-sndz launched at a price discount of 15% from the originator.[7] The initial price of infliximab-dyyb was 15% lower than the wholesale acquisition cost (WAC) of originator infliximab.[8] Since then, the second infliximab biosimilar, infliximab-abda, has launched at 35% discount off of WAC.[9] A similar trend has been documented in Europe. Although pricing discounts for certain products have reached the 70% to 80% threshold, smaller concessions in the 30% range are more common.[10,11]

While informative, these estimates are broad and fail to take into consideration the nuances of drug distribution and reimbursement as well as the various discounts and rebates that populate the U.S. pharmacy supply chain. To improve our ability to project value, we must first understand the variables that combine to affect the cost of pharmaceuticals, including biosimilars.

YOU ARE HERE!

The manufacturing steps and analytical characterization tools described in Chapters 3 and 4, respectively, may have appeared complex, but they pale in comparison to discerning the financial opportunity associated with biosimilars. Part of the challenge relates to differences in the way in which biologic medications are both distributed (traditional versus specialty distribution) and reimbursed (medical versus pharmacy benefit) across healthcare settings.[4,12] **Figure 10-1** illustrates the complexity of the U.S. healthcare system for pharmaceutical supply.[12-14] From a health-system pharmacy perspective, the right side of the graph may appear more familiar and that is where we will begin the discussion.

The Basics of Pharmacy Distribution

Drug manufacturers develop and produce medications.[14] By contrast, the work of providing an access point for most drugs primarily resides within the realm of pharmaceutical wholesalers/distributors.[14] These organizations take on the logistical challenge of obtaining medications across the multitude of pharmacy suppliers and delivering these products to retail and hospital pharmacies, physician offices, and other healthcare settings.[14] Over the course of time, the distribution environment has become increasingly consolidated where three primary companies now manage the majority of business nationally.[14] Most providers' routine drug purchases are through these organizations and/or their related subsidiaries.[14,15] The advent and growth of specialty pharmacy development has accompanied an increased focus on the ability to provide specialty pharmacy distribution services. Many new medications require additional monitoring, handling, and security and/or due to their expense are preferentially managed in a more narrow supply chain with product in limited locations.[15,16] This approach enables greater control of product and a decrease in the inventory on hand. Through both an expansion of capabilities of the three national primary distributors and other entities that participate primarily in the specialized space, specialty distribution has become an increasingly larger participant in the pharmacy supply chain.[15,16] This difference represents one of the initial issues that could affect the cost equation for biosimilars.

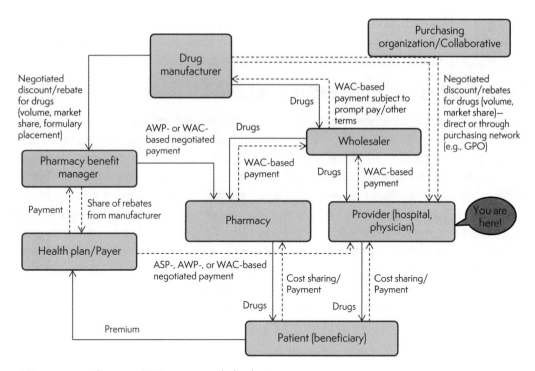

ASP = average sales price; AWP = average wholesale price;
GPO = group purchasing organization; WAC = wholesale acquisition cost

FIGURE 10-1. FLOW OF DRUGS AND PAYMENT IN THE U.S. HEALTHCARE SYSTEM.[12-14]

Cost Minus or Cost Plus

As seen in Figure 10-1, wholesalers obtain medication from manufacturers and in turn sell it to pharmacies and other providers. The WAC is a critical aspect of this transaction.[12] WAC is an industry term that denotes the list price paid for a prescription pharmaceutical that is available for sale by a manufacturer to a wholesaler.[12] However, manufacturers offer prompt pay terms such that if the wholesaler pays for their purchases in a designated timeframe (e.g., 30 days), they are in fact charged less than the WAC price.[12] In turn, wholesalers use these savings to offer volume-based discounts with their customers (e.g., hospital pharmacies).[12,17] This purchasing approach, frequently known by the term cost minus, means that hospital pharmacies purchase products from their wholesaler at a price lower than the initial list cost to wholesaler.[11,17-19] Products supplied through traditional distribution practices are usually subject to this discount. Unfortunately, this same methodology is not in place for specialty distribution as the management of these agents usually involves higher costs.[19] As cost minus opportunities are not available, there is no moderation of pricing associated with the initial acquisition of many expensive pharmaceuticals.[18,19] The selection of distribution channel, traditional or specialty, has been a source of increased scrutiny and some frustration over the last few years.[17-19] Several commonly-used branded biologics, including those that originally entered the market as regularly distributed products, have been moved to specialty distribution, thus increasing acquisition costs for hospitals and health systems.[17-19] As a result, one opportunity biosimilars have to differentiate themselves is the choice of traditional distribution if the originator currently manages its product through the specialty route. Conversely, the choice of specialty distribution for a biosimilar would likely represent a negatively viewed strategy from the provider point of view.

Group Purchasing Organizations and 340B

Another element that influences the purchase price of medications, particularly in the health-system setting, is the influence of collaborative purchasing agreements, such as those found through group purchasing organizations (GPOs).[13] GPOs leverage the collective purchasing power of multiple hospitals, health systems, and other practices to negotiate discounts for products.[13] In addition, GPOs help establish incentive programs with suppliers where additional discounts, or in some cases, rebates are provided for an increased volume of product purchased and/or a greater market share percentage for a pharmaceutical relative to other competing products.[13] GPOs and other collaborative purchasing arrangements represent another avenue by which biosimilar manufacturers can offer incentives, primarily to the acquisition price of a medication, to drive increased uptake relative to originator suppliers. If an originator supplier has previously not worked with GPOs to offer discounted pricing, this difference would represent another opportunity for a competing biosimilar to differentiate its value proposition.

An additional program that is critical to the competition for biosimilars is the influence of 340B pricing. The 340B program is part of the Public Health Service Act that allows certain organizations known as covered entities that provide care to various underserved populations to acquire outpatient pharmaceuticals at discounted prices.[20] The capacity of some providers and institutions to acquire and administer high-cost pharmaceuticals (i.e., branded biologics) is predicated on their ability to access 340B discounts.[20] As a result, for products expected to have a high usage pattern within covered entities, the provision of a competitive 340B price is another critical element to increase a biosimilar's viability compared to existing biologics.[4]

Beyond the initial price established for any product, including a biosimilar, the distribution channels, the influence of collaborative purchasing agreements, and availability of statutory pricing for eligible participants further influence actual acquisition cost. Pharmacists must remain cognizant of these variables within the total financial calculation of a biosimilar opportunity. Next we will examine an equally important part of calculating pharmaceutical value, the extent to which products are reimbursed.

COST VERSUS REIMBURSEMENT (MEDICAL VERSUS PHARMACY BENEFIT)

Another critical element to understanding the calculation of medication expenses is that the financial value of greatest interest is characterized in different ways depending on each stake-holder's role within the supply of pharmaceuticals.[12] For certain stakeholders, the acquisition cost of the medication is the most critical attribute.[4,12] In other circumstances, it is the difference or spread between cost and reimbursement that drives purchasing decisions.[4,12] This variation is likely best understood by contrasting medical and pharmacy benefits.

Within the world of healthcare insurance, medical benefits pertain to interventions that occur in a hospital or health-system setting.[12] Separately, pharmacy benefits involve coverages that support the acquisition of medications in the outpatient environment (e.g., retail pharmacy).[12] The related federal programs that most correlate to these designations are the Medicare categories of Part A (inpatient care), Part B (hospital outpatient or physician office care), and Part D (prescription drug benefit).[21] While not identical, the approach to reimbursement in these different settings is reasonably similar for private insurers.[12] Generic medications have historically fit into these various categories with limited overlap. For example, injectable medications, particularly critical care products reside within the acute care environment.[22] Similarly, infused products that do not require an inpatient admission have been administered by a healthcare provider in the hospital outpatient setting or physician office.[22,23] Finally, noninjectable medications, including many, blockbuster generics, have been provided through retail and mail-order pharmacies.[23] Unlike small molecule medications, biologics, particularly those targeted for biosimilar development, do not fall as easily into these clearly defined categories, but span multiple settings.[2,3] **Table 10-1** lists how drug costs and reimbursement vary across the different types of payment models.[4,12]

Within the context of an inpatient hospital visit, medications are generally not reimbursed separately.[12,21] As the choice of medication selected does not alter the overall reimbursement

TABLE 10-1. Financial Considerations for Drug Acquisition[4,12]

Stakeholder	Financial Considerations	How Drugs are Reimbursed	Implications for Biosimilars
Medical Benefit			
Hospitals (inpatient)	Cost	Drugs reimbursed as part of a bundle (e.g., diagnosis-related group [DRG] for Medicare); no separate payment	As pharmaceuticals are not reimbursed separately, the primary driver of value is related to cost minimization. Therefore, the lower cost product would be preferred.
Hospitals (outpatient), physician offices, clinic settings	Difference between cost and reimbursement	Drugs are reimbursed separately based on fee schedules related to a pricing benchmark such as average sales price (ASP), wholesale acquisition cost (WAC), or average wholesale price (AWP)	While lower cost products are important to minimize the acquisition expense of medications, reimbursement is critically significant as well. Given reimbursement methods, providers are currently incentivized to maximize the difference or spread between drug cost and amount reimbursed.
Pharmacy Benefit			
Pharmacy Benefit Manager (PBM)	Cost and incentive rebates/ discounts	Pharmacy benefit managers are interested in the acquisition cost as that drives the payment they make to pharmacies for dispensing medications. PBMs also negotiate with manufacturers to receive discounts and rebates for formulary placement of products and ability to influence market share and volume.	The cost of a biosimilar is important to this audience. The extent to which discounts and rebates can be obtained from the manufacturer is also important. This additional value is also important to the payer (insurer) as they may receive a negotiated portion of such rebates.

either through government (e.g., Medicare) or private insurers, the most cost-effective strategy for a hospital is to select clinically equivalent products with the lowest price. This strategy has driven the majority of cost considerations for hospitals through generic and therapeutic interchange programs.[12] In this setting, a biosimilar competing with a lower price relative to the originator reference product would likely be viewed favorably. Although not solely relegated to inpatient use, filgrastim has a substantial utilization presence in the acute care setting, which has contributed to some of the uptake seen with competing products like the separately licensed biologic, tbo-filgrastim, and the biosimilar filgrastim-sndz.[24] Outside of the hospital, different considerations influence purchasing patterns.

In the hospital outpatient and physician practice setting, medications that cost over a certain daily price threshold ($120 for 2018) are reimbursed separately.[12,25,26] Providers look not only to the acquisition price of the product, but also the extent of reimbursement. As a result, maximizing the difference between these two factors helps providers achieve their goal. The standard that is increasingly adopted to calculate reimbursement is the average sales price (ASP), introduced by the 2003 Medicare Prescription Drug, Improvement, and Modernization Act.[14] The ASP is calculated based on manufacturer reported actual selling price data and includes the majority of rebates, volume discounts, and other price concessions offered for a specific pharmaceutical.[12] This pricing information is submitted by manufacturers to Medicare. After a two-quarter delay, Medicare publishes an updated ASP.[12] Therefore, as prices increase or decrease, the ASP changes although in a delayed fashion.[12] For Medicare outpatient coverage (i.e., Part B), products currently administered in either the hospital outpatient or physician office setting are to be reimbursed 106% of the ASP for a medication.[12] It should be noted that due to budget sequestration that began in 2012 (and is currently scheduled to continue through 2025), the actual reimbursement rate is approximately 104.3% ASP.[27,28] Some insurers still use alternative metrics such as the average wholesale price (AWP), a sticker price that does not reflect the amount paid after pricing concessions; however, more have migrated to the ASP standard, although the percentage of add-on reimbursement may be higher than 6%.[12] In this circumstance, while lower product costs are desirable, they also have the negative effect of ultimately lowering the ASP calculation, which makes the creation of a differential value proposition more complicated.

THE INFLUENCE OF PHARMACY BENEFIT MANAGEMENT

The third aspect of medication delivery involves the dispensing of medications that do not necessarily have to be administered by a healthcare provider. This environment has historically been the realm of pharmacy benefit management (PBM) companies.[2] PBMs have been one of the greatest forces for driving the increased use of generics in the retail setting.[29] In this environment, the value equation differs still. The payer through a PBM determines which products are preferentially covered and available to the beneficiary/patient.[30] The cost that a PBM must pay a manufacturer for coverage of their product is very influential in establishing which medications will be included on the formulary.[2,12,30] PBMs negotiate discounts based on volume and market share criteria and also secure rebates from pharmaceutical manufacturers in exchange for preferential placement of medications on the approved formulary.[12] Many of the most commonly-used biologics that are targeted for biosimilar competition are self-injected medications like adalimumab and etanercept, which are covered under the pharmacy benefit.[30] Even before the advent of biosimilars, PBMs have established preferred lists for targeted drug categories, encouraging the use of molecularly distinct, yet therapeutically equivalent biologics.[2] For a biosimilar entrant, the value equation for this audience must include not just the price of the product, but also rebate considerations to establish preferential placement as compared to the originator.[12]

THE RISE OF SPECIALTY PHARMACY

As discussed in Chapter 1, biologics have played a prominent role in the growth of the specialty pharmacy industry.[2,3] The increased costs associated with biologics and specialty drugs have prompted efforts by both the provider audience and the payer environment to manage expense across all healthcare settings.[14,31] For example, while historically limited to true retail products, payers and PBMs have attempted to exert greater influence on products delivered in the outpatient infusion space through efforts such as *brown bagging* and *white bagging*.[15,31] These strategies differ from what is known as a traditional *buy and bill model*.[15,31]

In the *buy and bill* approach, a provider such as a hospital or physician office buys the medication, infuses it, and charges the patient/payer for both the cost of the pharmaceutical and its administration.[15] In contrast, *brown bagging* and *white bagging* are circumstances where the payer purchases the medication and through the coordination with a retail and/or specialty pharmacy delivers the patient-specific, labeled product to the either the patient (*brown bag*) or provider (*white bag*) for subsequent infusion.[15] In both of these situations, the provider can charge only for the administration of the product and not its purchase, a much lower revenue-generating opportunity.[15,16] Due in part to these efforts and given the increased responsibility to act as accountable care organizations, many health systems have initiated programs to establish internal specialty pharmacy capabilities.[31] Therefore, whether a payer implements a buy and bill methodology or white bagging strategy, the health system could ideally charge for the cost of the pharmaceutical and preserve continuity of care.[31]

Rather than being confined to one treatment setting and one set of purchasing and reimbursement rules, many biologics and by extension biosimilars extend across all of these sites of care. This change has and will continue to create challenges for biosimilars to define a proposition that is appealing to all audiences. It also establishes the potential for a misalignment of formulary coverage between a provider and the payer responsible for a patient's care. Pharmacists will have to evaluate these variances when determining the best product (or products) to select for their organization.

Biosimilar Reimbursement (in Theory)

In addition to a new pathway for approval, implementation of the Biologics Price Competition and Innovation Act also was accompanied by a new federal reimbursement methodology for biosimilars administered as outpatient medications (i.e., Medicare Part B). Under Medicare Part B, all medications are assigned a Healthcare Common Procedure Coding System (HCPCS) code.[12] Again, providers billing for reimbursement of an administered product currently receive 106% ASP (decreased to 104.3% ASP due to sequestration).[12,27] When generic competitors are introduced, those products, since they are identical to the originator branded product, share the same HCPCS code.[12] As the generic products are priced lower, the new ASP reflects the pricing of all agents (brand and generic). Thus, the ASP-associated reimbursement decreases.

The methodology for Medicare Part B biosimilar reimbursement is different. Rather than a biosimilar sharing a HCPCS code with an originator, biosimilars are assigned different codes.[4,32] Consequently, following the loss of exclusivity of a branded biologic, two HCPCS codes will exist, one for the originator and one for the biosimilar. Furthermore, biosimilars are to be reimbursed at 100% of the ASP for the biosimilar, plus 6% (currently 4.3% due to sequestration) of the ASP for the originator biologic.[4,32] As the originator biologic would be expected to remain more expensive, calculating the 6% off of the branded product's ASP is intended to encourage biosimilar adoption and lessen the tendency to use the more expensive branded originator.[4,32] Also, given that it takes time to monitor the pricing of a specific product, such as a newly launched biosimilar, the Centers for Medicare & Medicaid Services (CMS) has stated it will initially calculate reimbursement off of a biosimilar's WAC until the ASP can be established.[33] The details of this process are summarized in **Table 10-2**.

Biosimilar Reimbursement (First Approach)

As with many aspects of the biosimilar paradigm, this process for reimbursement did not address all questions concerning biosimilars. For example, while it was clear that biosimilars would not share the same HCPCS code of the originator reference product, an outstanding issue was whether biosimilars of the same branded agent would receive common or different codes. To some stakeholders' surprise, CMS initially ruled that biosimilars of the same originator reference product would share HCPCS codes.[34] This decision prompted concerns that the discounts offered by multiple biosimilar manufacturers to incentivize use of their products could more rapidly erode the shared ASP as compared to the reimbursement for the branded agent, thus

TABLE 10-2. Medicare Part B Reimbursement (Branded, Generic, and Biosimilar)[31,32,34]

Category	Medicare Part B Reimbursement
Branded drugs (small molecule and biologic)	■ Each individual agent receives a unique Healthcare Common Procedure Coding System (HCPCS) code ■ For both hospital outpatient and physician office (currently), reimbursement is 106% Average Sales Price (ASP) (or 104.3% ASP due to sequestration)
Generic small molecule drugs	■ Generic version shares same HCPCS code as the originator ■ ASP reflects pricing of the originator and generic; therefore, ASP declines as generic(s) enter the market at lower costs ■ Products reimbursed at 106% ASP (currently 104.3% ASP)
Biosimilars	■ Originator biologic keeps unique HCPCS code ■ All biosimilars now receive distinct HCPCS codes ■ Prior to the availability of adequate data to establish the ASP, biosimilars reimbursed according to their wholesale acquisition cost (WAC) ■ Biosimilar reimbursed at 100% of ASP for biosimilar and 6% of ASP for originator biologic (4.3% due to sequestration) ■ All biosimilars now eligible for "pass through" payment, which lasts two to three years

potentially making biosimilars less attractive to outpatient-based providers.[35] Another concern was that this decision of sharing HCPCS codes afforded the first biosimilar approved added leverage and authority. Under this interpretation, the first biosimilar would be reimbursed according to its WAC until enough pricing history is available to establish the true ASP.[34] Then, once the ASP would be set for a specific HCPCS code, all subsequent biosimilars of that same originator reference product would be reimbursed based on that amount.[36] As such, the second biosimilar would be reimbursed based on the pricing behavior of the initial marketed biosimilar.[36] In addition to this benefit, CMS decided that only the first approved biosimilar was eligible for additional pass-through payments to mitigate further the cost of new drug therapy.[36]

A Change in Strategy

A critical element that pharmacists must keep in mind is that reimbursement behaviors change over time. For example, private payers make changes to their formularies annually.[2] In addition, Medicare is continually adjusting factors such as the ASP as well as modifying other approaches.[21] As mentioned earlier in this chapter, CMS' reimbursement decisions have prompted concerns from both prospective biosimilar manufacturers and providers about the long-term viability of these products.[35] In its calendar year 2018 proposed Medicare Physician Fee Schedule, CMS had requested feedback regarding the impact of this decision.[37] Although CMS stated they were not committed to changing their approach, that is exactly what transpired.[38] With its finalization of the 2018 Physician Fee Schedule, CMS reversed its decision and begin assigning unique HCPCS codes to biosimilars of the same reference product.[38] The same approach will also be adopted for payment in the hospital outpatient setting.[39] As a result, the pricing decisions for each biosimilar manufacturer will only impact their individual ASP addressing concern about the cumulative discounts across multiple biosimilars. In addition, all biosimilars will now be eligible for pass-through payments.[39] Any biosimilar approved after January 1, 2018 will be reimbursed according to this process.[38,39] CMS has begun publishing detailed guidance regarding the change in coding for biosimilars that have been coded according to the previous model.[40,41] This change also adds another element for pharmacovigilance as each originator and associated biosimilar will have a unique identifier. CMS also stated that it will continue to monitor the biosimilar market and consider additional changes in the future.

MEDICARE PART D AND THE DONUT HOLE

The conversations regarding biosimilar reimbursement frequently involve health system-based or physician office-administered infused medications, agents that would be covered under Medicare Part B or the medical benefit of private insurers. Unfortunately, there is an outstanding issue concerning biosimilars and Medicare Part D.[42] As part of the Affordable Care Act, the government increased the discount manufacturers had to offer to help offset the expense of medications when patients fell into the donut hole (range preceding catastrophic coverage).[42] This program, the Coverage Gap Discount Program (CGDP), requires manufacturers to provide a 50% discount on brand drugs dispensed during this period of time.[42] This step helps ease the burden of patient acquisition costs for expensive medications. Unfortunately, this law only applies to branded drugs, not generics or biosimilars.[42] Under this current statute, Medicare Part D customers were not eligible for discounts from the biosimilar manufacturers during the time they were in the donut hole, which would make the patient expense greater as compared to use of a branded biologic.[42] The products primarily affected included those managed as outpatient, self-administered medications such as etanercept and adalimumab. Even though biosimilars for both products have been approved, their dates of launch are currently undefined given the uncertainty surrounding patent litigation issues.[43] However, as further evidence of the need to monitor regulatory decisions closely, this circumstance recently changed through the enactment of the Balanced Budget Act (BBA) of 2018.[44] Among many other provisions, the BBA made biosimilars eligible to participate in the CGDP, advanced the date for closure of the donut hole, and increased the percentage discount suppliers had to offer from 50% to 70%.[44,45] As a result, the inequity between coverage for biosimilars as compared to branded biologics appears to have been mitigated.

MEDICAID

Although much of our focus in the health-system landscape rests with Medicare, it is also important to understand the implications for biosimilars and Medicaid. The Medicaid program is sustained by the payment of rebates from pharmaceutical manufacturers.[12] The percentage of rebate paid is different depending on whether a product is a sole source (i.e., brand) or multi-source product.[12] CMS has reiterated its decision that while biosimilars are intended to compete with originator-branded products and create a multi-source experience, they are currently considered sole-source products.[46] Due to this decision, the rebates paid by biosimilar manufacturers will be at the higher percentage of 23.1% assigned to sole source products as compared to the 13% rebate of multi-source drugs.[46]

WHAT DOES THIS MEAN FOR PATIENTS?

Much of the conversation about biosimilars has centered on the extent to which savings will benefit the healthcare system overall or specifically groups such as payers or providers.[4,30] This concern is important as the increases in total healthcare expenditures appear excessive and unsustainable.[1,4] However, as healthcare providers, pharmacists must ensure that the impact to patients is not forgotten in the financial evaluations of value. If lower cost products come to market, but the financial hurdles to access care remain too high, patients will be unable to remain compliant, disease states will go untreated, and the healthcare market will bear the expense of higher cost, negative outcomes. Similarly, the potential exists for the payer community and the provider audience to take different approaches to biosimilar adoption.[4,30] This lack of alignment could make it more difficult for patients to obtain necessary treatment. Finally, one of the most critical elements of many aspects of medication access is the availability of patient assistance programs. Biosimilar manufacturers must provide support equal to if not greater than what is available through branded suppliers in terms of accessibility and utility.[30]

WHAT DOES THIS MEAN FOR PHARMACISTS?

The evaluation of financial benefit of biosimilars requires an appreciation of the complexity inherent in medication pricing, distribution, and reimbursement as well as the evolving nature of our healthcare systems. The calculation of financial opportunity will be more involved that what we have traditionally enjoyed with generic medications in the acute care environment. Rather than simply seeking the lowest priced alternative provided through our primary distribution avenue, we must also be cognizant of the decisions suppliers make regarding how they will distribute their biosimilars, what placement these products will have on the formularies of PBMs, and the impact pricing concessions and discounts have on reimbursement. Even after biosimilars are introduced, the profitability for originator products will still remain substantial for the branded manufacturer.[3] Therefore, we would expect the evaluation of economic value to remain an ongoing process as the brand and biosimilar suppliers compete for market share.[4] As such, financial stewardship in this era requires the continual monitoring of more economic variables than that to which we were previously accustomed. **Table 10-3** offers a checklist of key metrics pharmacists will need to consider to determine the greatest economic opportunity regarding biosimilars for their organizations and their patients.[12-21,38-40]

TABLE 10-3. Key Metrics for Assessing Biosimilar Value[12-21,31,32,34]

Cost	Reimbursement/Revenue
■ Wholesale acquisition cost	■ Reimbursement value of biosimilar compared to originator
■ Distribution channel (cost minus vs. cost plus)	• Average sales price based
■ Group purchasing organization contracts	• Average wholesale price based
• Standardization value	• Cost of charges
• Utilization value	■ Part B versus Part D coverage
■ Direct agreements from originator or biosimilar manufacturer	■ Coverage determinations for private payers
■ 340B pricing	• Preferred placement
■ Availability and accessibility of patient assistance programs	• White bag/brown bag strategies
	■ Other
	• Pass-through payments from CMS for all biosimilars

CMS = Centers for Medicare & Medicaid Services.

KEY POINTS

- The mechanisms for the purchase, distribution, and reimbursement of medications are very complicated and difficult to understand.

- The introduction of a completely new class of medications (i.e., biosimilars) will only add to that level of complexity.

- While challenging, pharmacists must be willing to scrutinize all of the factors that influence the cost and reimbursement of medications to assess to what extent biosimilars might offer meaningful value for both their organizations and to the patients for whom they provide care.

- Pharmacists must remain vigilant for continual changes to the cost and reimbursement landscape.

CONCLUSION

Biosimilars will not exist in the absence of a financially compelling justification for their use. The determination of what degree of value is meaningful will vary across different stakeholders and will change over the continued development of biosimilars. Pharmacists must understand all of the factors that converge to determine the true financial value for biosimilars. In addition, they must be sensitive to the way in which other parts of their organizations or even other participants in the healthcare landscape view the economic incentives to using biosimilars and how those financial decisions impact the patient.

REFERENCES

1. McCamish M, Woollett G. Worldwide experience with biosimilar development. *mAbs.* 2011;3(2):209-17.

2. Falit BP, Singh SC, Brennan TA. Biosimilar competition in the United States: statutory incentives, payers, and pharmacy benefit managers. *Health Aff (Millwood).* 2015;34:294-301.

3. Blackstone EA, Fuhr JP. The economics of biosimilars. *Am Health Drug Benefits.* 2013;6:469-78.

4. Mulcahy AW, Predmore Z, Mattke S. The cost savings potential of biosimilar drugs in the United States. www.rand.org/content/dam/rand/pubs/perspectives/PE100/PE127/RAND_PE127.pdf (accessed Mar. 20, 2018).

5. DiMasi JA, Grabowski HG, Hansen RW. Innovation in the pharmaceutical industry: new estimates of R & D costs. *J Health Econ.* 2016;47:20-33.

6. IMS Health. Shaping the biosimilars opportunity: a global perspective on the evolving biosimilars landscape. www.weinberggroup.com/pdfs/Shaping_the_biosimiliars_opportunity_A_global_perspective_on_the_evolving_biosimiliars_landscape.pdf (accessed Mar. 20, 2018).

7. Johnson SR. One year after Zarxio approval, future of biosimilars remains unclear. www.modern-healthcare.com/article/20160323/NEWS/160319919 (accessed Mar. 20, 2018).

8. Pfizer announces the U.S. availability of biosimilar INFLECTRA® (infliximab-dyyb). Press release. www.pfizer.com/news/press-release/press-release-detail/pfizer_announces_the_u_s_availability_of_biosimilar_inflectra_infliximab_dyyb (accessed Mar. 20, 2018).

9. Sagonowsky E. Targeting a $5B brand, Samsung and Merck launch Remicade biosim at 35% discount. http://www.fiercepharma.com/pharma/samsung-merck-launch-remicade-biosim-at-35-discount. (accessed Mar. 20, 2018).

10. Asbjorn M. Norway, biosimilars in different funding systems. What works? www.gabi-journal.net/norway-biosimilars-in-different-funding-systems-what-works.html (accessed Mar. 20, 2018).

11. Delivering on the Potential of Biosimilar Medicines: The Role of Functioning Competitive Markets. IMS Health, March 2016. www.iqvia.com/-/media/iqvia/pdfs/institute-reports/delivering-on-the-potential-of-biosimilar-medicines.pdf?la=en&hash=7705453CF0E82E-F41402A87A44744FBF8D84327C&_=1521578497886 (accessed Mar. 20, 2018).

12. AMCP Guide to Pharmaceutical Payment Methods, 2013 Update, version 3.0. http://www.amcp.org/pharmaceutical-payment-guide/ (accessed Mar. 20, 2018).

13. ASHP guidelines on medication cost management strategies for hospitals and health systems. *Am J Health Syst Pharm.* 2008;65:1368-84.

14. Avalere Health. Follow the Pill: understanding the U.S. Commercial Pharmaceutical Supply Chain. March 2005. http://avalere.com/research/docs/Follow_the_Pill.pdf (accessed Mar. 20, 2018).

15. McCain J. Connecting patients with specialty products, part 1: distribution models for biologics and other specialty pharmaceutical products. *Biotechnol Healthc.* 2012;9:8-13.

16. McCain J. Connecting patients with specialty products, Part 2: the future of specialty drug distribution. *Biotechnol Healthc.* 2012;9:13-6.

17. Saporito B. Hospitals furious at cancer-drug price hikes. *Time*. October 27, 2014. http://time.com/3541484/cancer-drug-price-hikes/ (accessed Mar. 20, 2018).

18. Thompson CA. Not all discounts on certain cancer drugs have disappeared. *Am J Health Syst Pharm*. 2015;72:259-60.

19. Traynor K. Pharmacists pan Genentech distribution model. *Am J Health Syst Pharm*. 2015;72:6-7.

20. Kantarjian H, Chapman R. The 340B drug pricing program: background, concerns, and solutions. www.ascopost.com/issues/january-25-2016/the-340b-drug-pricing-program-background-concerns-and-solutions/ (accessed Mar. 20, 2018).

21. Danzon PM. Pricing and reimbursement of biopharmaceuticals and medical devices in the USA. In: *Encyclopedia of Health Economics*. New York: Elsevier;2014: 127-35.

22. Schumock GT, Li ED, Wiest MD, et al. National trends in prescription drug expenditures and projections for 2017. *Am J Health Syst Pharm*. 2017;74:1158-73.

23. QuintilesIMS. Medicines Use and Spending in the U.S., a review of 2016 and outlook to 2021. May 2017. http://www.imshealth.com/en/thought-leadership/quintilesims-institute/reports/medicines-use-and-spending-in-the-us-review-of-2016-outlook-to-2021 (accessed Mar. 20, 2018).

24. Traynor K. Filgrastim becomes biosimilar test case for hospitals. *Am J Health Syst Pharm*. 2016;73:1805-6.

25. Kirschenbaum B. Reimbursement matters: Vital conversations to have with your finance team. Pharmacy Practice News. www.pharmacypracticenews.com/Article/PrintArticle?articleID=37851 (accessed Mar. 20, 2018).

26. Kirschenbaum, B. OPPS proposed 2018 rules: effects on pharmacy. Pharmacy Practice News. www.pharmacypracticenews.com/Article/PrintArticle?articleID=44568 (accessed Mar. 17, 2018).

27. Polite BN, Ward JC, Cox JV, et al. Payment for oncolytics in the United States: a history of buy and bill and proposals for reform. *J Oncol Pract*. 2014;10:357-62.

28. Luthi S. CHIP, Medicare extenders caught in battle over sequester. www.modernhealthcare.com/article/20171201/NEWS/171209979. (accessed Mar. 20, 2018).

29. Asclone FJ, Kirking DM, Gaither CA, Welage LS. Historical overview of generic medication policy. *J Am Pharm Assoc*. 2001;41:567-77.

30. Rumore MM, Vogenberg F.Biosimilars: still not quite ready for prime time. *PT*.2016;41:366-75.

31. ASHP Specialty Pharmacy Resource Guide. https://www.ashp.org/-/media/assets/pharmacy-practice/resource-centers/specialty-pharmacy/specialty-pharmacy-resource-guide.ashx?la=en (accessed Mar. 20, 2018).

32. Wynne B. Implementation of the biosimilars provisions of the ACA—where are we now? http://healthaffairs.org/blog/2015/12/14/implementation-of-the-biosimilars-provisions-of-the-aca-where-are-we-now/. (accessed Mar. 20, 2018).

33. Food and Drug Administration Approval of First Biosimilar Product. MLN Matters. https://www.cms.gov/Outreach-and-Education/Medicare-Learning-Network-MLN/MLNMattersArticles/Downloads/SE1509.pdf (accessed Mar. 20, 2018).

34. Xcenda. CMS proposes to bundle biosimilars into single ASP per reference product. http://www.xcenda.com/Insights-Library/Archive/CMS-Proposes-to-Bundle-Biosimilars-Into-Single-ASP-per-Reference-Product/ (accessed Mar. 20, 2018).

35. Biosimilars forum disappointed with CMS final rule on biosimilar payment and coding. Biosimilars Forum press release. www.biosimilarsforum.org/news/biosimilars-forum-disappointed-cms-final-rule-biosimilar-payment-and-coding (accessed Mar. 20, 2018).

36. CY2016 Hospital Outpatient Prospective Payment System. *Federal Register*. 2015 (November 13); 80 (219). www.gpo.gov/fdsys/pkg/FR-2015-11-13/pdf/2015-27943.pdf (accessed Mar. 20, 2018).

37. Department of Health and Human Services. Centers for Medicare & Medicaid Services. Medicare Programs; Revisions to payment policies under the Physician Fee Schedule and Other Revisions to Part B for CY 2018. https://s3.amazonaws.com/public-inspection.federalregister.gov/2017-14639.pdf (accessed Mar. 20, 2018).

38. Department of Health and Human Services. Centers for Medicare & Medicaid Services. 42 CFR Parts 405, 410, 414, 424, and 425. Medicare Program; Revisions to payment policies under the Physician Fee Schedule and Other Revisions to Part B for CY 2018; Medicare Shared Savings Program Requirements; and Medicare Diabetes Prevention Program. https://s3.amazonaws.com/public-inspection.federalregister.gov/2017-23953.pdf (accessed Mar. 20,2018).

39. Department of Health and Human Services. Centers for Medicare & Medicaid Services. 42 CFR Parts 414, 416, and 419. Medicare Program: Hospital Outpatient Prospective Payment and Ambulatory Surgical Center Payment Systems and Quality Reporting Programs. https://s3.amazonaws.com/public-inspection.federalregister.gov/2017-23932.pdf (accessed Mar. 20, 2018).

40. Syrop J. CMS reverses its policy on biosimilar reimbursement, will issue unique J-codes. http://www.centerforbiosimilars.com/news/cms-reverses-its-policy-on-biosimilars-reimbursement-will-issue-unique-jcodes. (accessed Mar. 20, 2018).

41. Centers for Medicare and Medicaid Services. Part B biosimilar biological product payment and required modifiers. https://www.cms.gov/Medicare/Medicare-Fee-for-Service-Part-B-Drugs/McrPartBDrugAvgSalesPrice/Part-B-Biosimilar-Biological-Product-Payment.html. (accessed Mar. 17, 2018).

42. Patient out-of-pocket costs for biosimilars in Medicare Part D. Avalere Health, April 2016. http://go.avalere.com/acton/attachment/12909/f-02c0/1/-/-/-/-/20160412_Patient%20OOP%20for%20Biosimilars%20in%20Part%20D.pdf (accessed Mar. 20, 2018).

43. Kane A. FDA approves third biosimilar for arthritis—Amjevita, a biosimilar to Humira. http://blog.arthritis.org/news/humira-arthritis-biosimilar-fda-approved/. (accessed Mar. 20, 2018).

44. Burke SP, Rao A, Sadle SE. Key health care provisions of Bipartisan Budget Act of 2018. www.lexology.com/library/detail.aspx?g=e3315f80-731d-488a-885c-1fb42724fc67 (accessed Mar. 17, 2018).

45. McCaughan M. The budget blindside: did Pharma fight the wrong battle? *The Pink Sheet*, Feb. 21, 2018 (accessed Mar. 17, 2018).

46. Kelly C. Biosimilars ineligible for reduced Medicaid rebates as authorized generics. *The Pink Sheet*, Jan. 3, 2017 (accessed Mar. 17, 2018).

CHAPTER 11

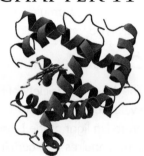

Biosimilar Formulary Management Strategies

The previous chapters in this text have described the manufacturing principles, the approval pathways, and the legal and financial hurdles that affect the launch of a biosimilar. After all of these steps and considerations have taken place, healthcare organizations, prescribers, and payers must still commit to the use of these products and do the work needed to support conversion and adoption. Unlike generic medications whose introduction is facilitated by a higher degree of familiarity as well as the commonality of key identifiers and attributes (e.g., same nonproprietary naming, therapeutic equivalency ratings), biosimilars will be accompanied by more operational differences.[1,2] Although biosimilars require some measure of formulary review prior to introduction, this process is different than the evaluation of new molecular entities.[3] Rather than an exhaustive analysis of clinical trial data, a biosimilar review should address a range of practice and information management issues to ensure safety and clarity of product use.[4] This chapter examines those issues as well as the level of supporting education needed to facilitate the transition to biosimilars once such products are added to organizations' formularies.

SIMILAR PRODUCTS, DIFFERENT FORMULARY REVIEW

Defined best practice recommendations state that a formulary review is not necessary for most generic medications given the fact that these products are identical to their reference counterparts.[5] Conversely, a formulary analysis is needed for evaluation of a novel molecular entity.[5] Biosimilars occupy a third, "gray" area of being neither absolutely identical, nor completely distinct molecularly. While a review is required, it is unique from the one with which most clinicians are familiar. For example, a biosimilar licensed by the Food and Drug Administration (FDA) will have met the threshold of high similarity with no clinically meaningful differences in safety, purity, and potency.[2,6] As a result, an intense scrutiny of clinical, pharmacodynamic, pharmacokinetic, and pharmacologic data is likely of limited utility since approval of a biosimilar signifies the product has already matched the parameters and attributes of the originator to FDA's satisfaction.[6] Obviously, substantial education, particularly of physicians, will be required to reinforce this perspective to ensure successful formulary management.

In contrast, an issue that might necessitate even greater review than that of a novel molecule is the concern regarding potential confusion related to the naming and dosage forms of the biosimilar.[1,3] Pharmacists are taught to monitor and avoid look-alike and sound-alike issues between medications.[5] However, commonality of a biosimilar to the originator biologic is the desired perception as such products are intended to perform just like the branded version. Still, differentiation remains an important issue for not only clinical, but also financial considerations.

As such, the formulary review process involves an exercise in identifying the points where similarity is no longer desired, but is potentially problematic.

Critical Elements of a Biosimilar Formulary Document

The American Society of Health-System Pharmacists (ASHP) has defined the elements of a drug evaluation document to support a formulary review.[5] In **Table 11-1**, those elements are interpreted in light of the biosimilar evaluation process. As is enumerated, the definition of biosimilarity requires that certain elements be the same between the biosimilar and the brand likely minimizing the need for scrutiny. Conversely, the similarity of other attributes prompts the need for more thorough evaluation and dialogue.

TABLE 11-1. Elements of a Drug-Evaluation Document to Support a Biosimilar Evaluation[1,3,4,6-12]

Element	Variation Between Biosimilar and Branded	Comment
Brand and generic (i.e., nonproprietary) names and synonyms	Different	■ Names, both brand and nonproprietary, will be different between biosimilar and originator reference product. ■ Pharmacovigilance and minimization of medication errors necessitates accurate identification of biosimilar and reference product.
FDA approval information, including date and FDA rating	Different	■ Important as all follow-on biologics are not necessarily biosimilars. ■ Product could be a true biosimilar, 351(k) licensed biosimilar (e.g., filgrastim-sndz); separately licensed 351(a) biologic (e.g., tbo-filgrastim); or 505b(2) product (e.g., insulin glargine). ■ Approval process can influence indication coverage; 351(k) products eligible for indication extrapolation, but not 351(a) approved biologics.
Pharmacology and mechanism of action	Same	■ By definition, the pharmacology and mechanism of action, to the extent it is known, must be the same between the originator reference product and the biosimilar.
FDA-approved indications	Same, but may not include entire complement of originator indications	■ The biosimilar is limited to indications for which the originator reference product is licensed. ■ The biosimilar applicant may not receive approval for all originator indications (e.g., orphan indication exclusivity) or may choose only to pursue certain indications.

(continued)

TABLE 11-1. (Continued)

Element	Variation Between Biosimilar and Branded	Comment
Potential non-FDA-approved (off-label) uses	Same	■ It should be clear to pharmacists and prescribers, which indications, if any, are not included in the biosimilar's label (due to factors such as orphan exclusivity for the brand). ■ External data may exist for biosimilar safety and efficacy for other indications for which the product is not currently licensed.
Dosage forms and storage	Possibly different	■ For certain biologics, particularly those that are self-administered, the dosage form presentation is patented; as a result, the biosimilar will be in a distinct presentation, prompting a need for appropriate patient education. ■ For healthcare provider administered products, differences may also exist if biosimilar does not pursue all presentations of the originator. ■ Also, there may be differences (both positive and negative) for storage requirements and shelf-life between biosimilar and originator.
Recommended dosage regimens	Same	■ The strength, potency, dosage, frequency of the biosimilar must be the same as the originator reference product.
Pharmacokinetic considerations	Same	■ Biosimilar evaluation includes pharmacokinetic studies, which must meet the standard of high similarity.
Use in special populations (e.g. children, elderly, patients with renal or liver failure)	Same	■ The standard of high similarity means that the biosimilar would be expected to work in the same way in special populations as the originator reference product; in addition, the guidance on labeling suggests that the considerations for the biosimilar in special populations will be the same as that of the originator.
Pregnancy category and use during breast-feeding	Same	■ See above comment for "special populations."

(continued)

TABLE 11-1. (Continued)

Element	Variation Between Biosimilar and Branded	Comment
Comparisons of the drug's efficacy, safety, convenience, and costs with those of therapeutic alternatives (with evidence tables when feasible)	Efficacy, safety (same)	■ To meet the standard of biosimilarity, the approved product must not have any clinically meaningful differences in terms of safety, purity, and potency. Also, clinical studies that support biosimilarity are intended to demonstrate comparability, not separately validate clinical efficacy.
	Convenience (possibly different)	■ As stated above, to compete effectively, the biosimilar must be as easy to use as the originator.
	Cost (different)	■ The purpose of the biosimilar paradigm is to introduce competition and lower costs for biologics. A formulary evaluation will likely center on this aspect. More detail on this consideration is provided in Chapter 10.
If information on comparative efficacy is minimal or lacking, data on absolute efficacy (i.e., efficacy versus placebo)	Different	■ In 351 (k) biosimilar trials, the comparisons are always against an active comparator (i.e., the originator).
Clinical trial analysis and critique	Different	■ The purpose of the clinical trials of a biosimilar is different. The intent is to establish similarity of the products, not independently prove safety and efficacy of the molecule. ■ The clinical endpoints between the clinical trials of the originator and the clinical data for the biosimilar could be different. ■ Clinical data will be more targeted and leverage the benefit of extrapolation and bridging. ■ FDA will have already concluded that the clinical data are sufficient to demonstrate biosimilarity.

(continued)

TABLE 11-1. (Continued)

Element	Variation Between Biosimilar and Branded	Comment
Medication safety assessment and recommendations (adverse drug reactions; drug-drug and drug-food interactions; specific therapy monitoring requirements; unusual administration; storage or stability issues; and potential for medication errors, such as look-alike/sound-alike issues)	Medication safety (same) Medication error potential (different)	■ The biosimilar will be labeled with the same considerations for adverse drug events, drug-drug and drug-food interactions, etc. ■ The differences in nomenclature will potentially present challenges, especially as it relates to duplication of therapy. ■ Must ensure thorough review for sound-alike/look-alike issues in relation to use of the biosimilar and the originator, especially if both products remain on formulary.
Financial analysis, including pharmacoeconomic analysis	Different	■ The availability of the biosimilar is intended to introduce competition and lower costs. Analyses should take into consideration both acquisition cost and reimbursement not only for the provider, but also for the patient. Additional information on this subject is provided in Chapter 10.

Which Elements Are the Same?

As can be seen from above, the biosimilar formulary review process is by no means unimportant. It is simply a slightly different focus. For example, by statutory definition and regulatory guidance a biosimilar must possess the same mechanism of action and pharmacology (to the extent that such elements are known), the same dosage range, and the same strength as the originator.[6,9] The information regarding special populations and pregnancy category considerations will likely be very similar since these instructions are based on the knowledge established for the originator reference product.[6,11] The commonality of labeling (i.e., package insert information) was further established in FDA's biosimilar labeling guidance.[11] Also, the scope of the labeled indications for biosimilars is limited to the uses for which the originator is approved.[9] Biosimilars may not necessarily be approved for all indications of the originator depending on which uses a manufacturer chooses to pursue and which indications retain certain protections (e.g., orphan drug exclusivity).[6,9] Similarly, a biosimilar is restricted from pursuing an indication for which the branded biologic does not have coverage.[2,6,9] Given the commonality of many of these attributes, devoting a significant time to their scrutiny is not required.

Which Elements Are Different?

The Role of Clinical Data

As stressed in Chapter 7, it is critically important that pharmacists, physicians, and other prescribers not lose sight of the intended purpose of clinical trial data in biosimilar approvals. Clinical trial information for novel biologics and biosimilars serve different purposes.[6,11,12] While they both help assess the safety and efficacy of the products studied, the way in which they achieve this goal is different. For a completely new medication, the safety and efficacy profile must be established in its entirety.[12] In contrast, the capabilities of analytical characterization and nonclinical, pharmacokinetic, and pharmacodynamic information minimize the degree of clinical data needed to confirm biosimilarity, validate the absence of performance differences, and address any residual uncertainties.[12] The size of a biosimilar trial, the population selected for study, and the indication(s) investigated could all vary from previously conducted clinical analyses of the originator.[6,10] Also, the scientifically justified principle of extrapolation further diminishes the need for replication of redundant clinical trial data across different indications.[12] As a result, formulary analyses should not focus on matching the structure and/or quantity of clinical data from a biosimilar study with previously conducted trials of the originator biologic. Pharmacists and physicians must understand the *totality of the evidence* approach employed by FDA to incorporate all submitted data, including clinical trial information, into a comprehensive picture that establishes biosimilarity.

Product Naming

As described in Chapter 7, FDA has finalized its guidance for the nonproprietary naming of biologics. All recombinant biologic drugs, including biosimilars, will have unique a nonproprietary *proper name* that includes a four-letter, devoid of meaning, suffix (e.g., infliximab-dyyb).[1,7] While the suffix is intended to allow the differentiation of a biosimilar with its originator, both products will continue to share the *core name* component (e.g., infliximab). As a result, there will definitely be look-alike and sound-alike considerations. We have seen and expect the continuation of suppliers assigning proprietary names to biosimilars.[13] The formulary review should address how this combination of nomenclature conveys the similarity of safety and efficacy to the branded product, and also allows for differentiation of the biosimilar ensuring safe prescribing and appropriate pharmacovigilance. This variation has numerous implications for the use of order entry, inventory management, and medication administration documentation processes and all information systems that support these activities.[1,3,4]

Approval Processes

The approval processes for originator and biosimilars are different.[1] In addition, not all follow-on biologics will necessarily receive approval through the biosimilars pathway. As described in Chapter 6, novel biologics are licensed through the 351(a) pathway and biosimilars through the 351(k).[4] However, tbo-filgrastim while approved as a biosimilar globally, received licensing through the 351(a) pathway in the United States.[4] This difference affects multiple aspects of this product's approval including its extent of indication coverage and exclusion from any subsequent considerations regarding interchangeability.[1] Also, certain recombinant biologics like the insulin analogs were originally approved through New Drug Applications rather than Biologics License Applications.[14] Until March 2020, follow-on versions of products such as glargine will likely be licensed via the 505b(2) pathway.[2,14] These agents are not currently considered biosimilars.

Differences in Dosage Forms

A crucial element for healthcare providers and patients alike is the potential for variation in the dosage forms of biosimilars.[3,10] Although a biosimilar must match the strength and dose of an originator counterpart, its approval is not contingent on replicating every formulation of the branded version.[6,9] This variation has come to light with initial biologic competition in the filgrastim market, both with the separately licensed tbo-filgrastim and the true biosimilar, filgrastim-sndz. Both of these agents came to market with pre-filled syringe presentations.[15,16] Unfortunately, neither manufacturer chose to pursue vial presentations on initial product launch, creating challenges for patients requiring tailored doses (e.g., pediatric populations).[17] Consequently, organizations with a large pediatric population may not find these products as viable alternatives to the brand. As articulated in Chapter 9, certain dosage forms such as the autoinjector products are patent protected.[10] Due to this exclusivity consideration, a biosimilar autoinjector will be different. This difference potentially causes issues related to storage and creates demands for awareness, training, and education for health care providers and patients alike.[3,10]

Inventory Management

The presence of similar products that vary in terms of naming, labeling, and formulation presents numerous challenges for efficient and safe inventory management, particularly if organizations must maintain both the originator and the biosimilar in stock. Pharmacists will need to consider if formulation availability, labeled indications, pricing, and reimbursement coverage allow the use of only one product.[1,3,4] If not, safety considerations must be in place throughout the ordering, storage, preparation, and delivery/dispensing processes for these products to prevent confusion in prescribing and administration.[1,3,4]

Expense of Conversion

Although issues such as naming, labeling, and presentations developed will be different for biosimilars, the biggest variation should be an economic one. Chapter 10 referenced many aspects of the biosimilar economic model that will impact acquisition cost and reimbursement. However, there is another expense that must be considered, the cost of conversion. For all of the elements listed above, pharmacists and technicians will have to invest time and dedication to ensure accuracy in drug ordering, preparation, delivery, administration, and monitoring when incorporating a biosimilar into practice.[1,3,4] **Table 11-2** lists some of these elements that should be factored into a conversion analysis. Pharmacists must ensure all other stakeholders who are involved in medication management are fully educated and comfortable in their understanding of biosimilars.[1,3,4]

Formulary Guidelines and Therapeutic Interchange

The entirety of the intent of the biosimilar pathway is to license products expected to behave just like their originator reference counterparts, which can be prescribed for the same situations and circumstances as the originator brands.[2] Direct acceptance of that perspective may not occur immediately, particularly when considering the use of biosimilars in patients who have already initiated therapy with the originator reference product.[1,10] Pharmacists will have to assist their

TABLE 11-2. Other Cost Considerations for Biosimilars[1,3,4]

Conversion cost	■ What is the cost of transitioning to the biosimilar?
	■ How much physician, pharmacist, and nursing education will be required to support successful launch and adoption?
	■ How much patient education will be required to answer all questions concerning safety, efficacy, and cost?
	■ What is the cost of changing products across all databases in all clinical information, production, compounding, inventory, and financial management systems?
	■ What is the cost of changing to a different formulation, if not all presentations are available?

organizations in determining to what extent a biosimilar is accepted as substitutable or therapeutically interchangeable with the brand.[1,10]

As discussed in Chapter 6, the formal FDA designation of interchangeability has yet to be conferred on any licensed biosimilar and still remains a concept under development.[10] The underlying principle is that a patient can be switched safety back and forth between the interchangeable biologic and the originator with no greater risk of adverse events or negative clinical outcomes than if the therapy were maintained with the branded product all along.[10] Until such time as the interchangeability designation is actually granted, pharmacists will have to work with their physicians to agree as to what extent and in which populations can the biosimilar be used in place of the branded biologic (e.g., naïve or non-naïve).[1,3,4,10] Whether the decision is complete replacement of the branded product with the biosimilar or use of multiple versions of the same biologic, pharmacists will have to ensure that such a decision is clearly delineated for physicians, nurses, and all care providers.[3,4] Even for organizations that select a process that does not require universal brand replacement, effective use of biosimilars can be facilitated through the therapeutic interchange programs that have existed for molecularly distinct products such as the erythropoietins (epoetin versus darbepoetin) and the intravenous immune globulins.[4]

Finally, any formulary decision, whether involving a complete or only partial substitution of a biosimilar for its branded comparator, must include a defined methodology for pharmacovigilance.[3,10] Again, given the rigor of the FDA approval process and the experiences established within Europe and other highly-regulated markets, we would not expect a higher adverse event rate or inferior clinical outcomes with biosimilars.[4,12] Still, collecting such data on both the biosimilar and the originator reference product can help allay concerns by further establishing the comparability of clinical effects. In addition, a prominent need and area of focus within healthcare is the goal of correlating outcomes with various interventions, including pharmaceuticals. Improved pharmacovigilance enables the characterization of benefits and risks associated with all medications, hopefully to the point where product costs will more directly align with patient outcomes.

EDUCATION

Physician Education

A critical educational requirement related to biosimilars and their successful adoption is the understanding and awareness of the prescriber community. If physicians do not embrace the principles of biosimilarity or accept their qualifications as products of equal safety and efficacy as compared to originator biologics, the biosimilar model will not be successful. Fortunately, the approval and introduction of products has appeared to increase the overall awareness and, in some cases, acceptance of biosimilars. For example, an often-referenced 2011 survey of oncology practitioners revealed that 39% of pharmacists, 64% of nurses, and 58% of physicians were only slightly familiar or not at all familiar with developments in biosimilars.[18] We must recognize that at the point in time of the survey, the Biologics Price Competition and Innovation Act was only one year into existence, no guidance information had yet been published, and no biosimilars had received approval.[2,13,18] Given the continued progress in product introduction, subsequent assessments have reflected differing trends.

The Biosimilars Forum, an advocacy organization of 10 manufacturers who are in the process of developing biosimilars, recently published the results of a survey of specialty physicians conducted between November 2015 and January 2016.[19] The survey included 19 questions intended to assess the level of awareness, knowledge, and perceptions of biosimilars among U.S. specialty physicians who already prescribe biologics. Survey responses were obtained from 1,201 U.S. specialty physicians including dermatologists, gastroenterologists, hematologist-oncologists, medical oncologists, nephrologists, and rheumatologists. The results demonstrate variations across specialties. For example, almost 50% of most of the specialties correctly responded that biosimilars had just become available in the United States during the previous year, yet only 34.5% of rheumatologists answered this question correctly.[19] In addition, over 55% of rheumatologists responded incorrectly that no biosimilars were available.[19] These responses should not be used to single out any particular specialty. Instead, these findings should encourage the continued discussion about biosimilar developments with all prescribers, even those not yet directly affected by the introduction of these agents. For example, the only biosimilar approved at the time of this survey was filgrastim-sndz, an oncology-related agent.[13] In the eight months following this survey, three more products used in inflammatory diseases (infliximab-dyyb, etanercept-szzs, and adalimumab-atto) were approved.[13] Clearly, a specialty area with limited exposure to biosimilars can quickly transition to one confronted with multiple related products.

The hallmark of biosimilars is that the approved products will have no clinically meaningful differences in terms of safety, purity, or potency.[2,6] According to the survey, 62.3% of all respondents agreed with the statement that a biosimilar will have equivalent efficacy as its originator brand counterpart.[19] In addition, 57.2% agreed that a biosimilar will be at least as safe as the originator brand.[19] While these numbers reflect an increasing level of comprehension, almost 40% of specialty physicians were not fully versed and accepting of the primary concept of a biosimilarity determination.[19] In addition, 35.9% of respondents stated that biosimilars are less safe than the originator biologic because the approval pathway is abbreviated.[19] Even though the level of awareness continues to increase, a substantial percentage of prescribers who will interact with these agents do not clearly understand many essential details of the biosimilar paradigm.

As discussed in previous chapters, the European Union has confronted many similar issues given the longer duration of experience it has had with biosimilars. This perspective applies to physician education and comprehension about biosimilars. The European Crohn's and Colitis Organization recently published the results of a survey of its members intended as an update from one conducted in 2013.[20] The responses to the updated questionnaire demonstrated a higher degree of acceptance and comfort with biosimilars.[20] For example, in 2013, 67.1% of respondents believed that there would be higher immunogenicity with biosimilars and 43.1% felt that biosimilars would have a different mechanism of action as compared to the originator.[20] In the 2015 survey, the numbers had decreased to 27.1% concerned about immunogenicity and 16.9% who felt biosimilars would have a different action.[20] Furthermore, the number of respondents who were totally confident or very confident in biosimilars increased from 12.6% in 2013 to 46.6% in 2015.[20] Additional use and increasing familiarity with these agents helps to moderate preexisting concerns.

Areas recommended for focus of physician education include the following:[19]

- Defining biologics, biosimilars, and biosimilarity
- Understanding the approval process and the use of "totality of evidence" to evaluate biosimilars
- Understanding that the safety and immunogenicity of a biosimilar are comparable to the originator biologics
- Understanding the rationale for extrapolation of indications
- Defining interchangeability and the related rules regarding pharmacy-level substitution

Although physicians stand at the top of the list of stakeholders requiring more in depth education, pharmacists must similarly include nurses and other clinicians in training on the biosimilarity concept.

Patient Education

While successful adoption of biosimilars cannot occur in the absence of physician understanding and approval, meaningful use of these products will fail to succeed without the comfort and commitment of the patient community. This need for acceptance was illustrated recently in an international survey sponsored by Pfizer, a biosimilars' developer.[21] The on-line survey included 3,198 respondents from the United States and European Union including diagnosed patients with certain inflammatory or oncology diseases, diagnosed patients who participated in advocacy/support groups, caregivers of patients with these diseases, and representatives of the general population.[21] The survey revealed that the overall awareness of biosimilars was low—6%—in the general population; while numerically higher, the general awareness of biosimilars in the diagnosed population was still very low at 9%.[21] Patients who not only had disease, but also who had participated in support groups reported a 20%-level of awareness.[21] Awareness may not encapsulate a complete appreciation of all elements of the biosimilarity discussion, but it can influence patients' willingness to consider use of these agents. For example, when comparing patients who were at least aware of biosimilars versus those who were not, 17% more felt comfortable switching to a biosimilar, 17% more agreed such products were safe, and 18% more agreed biosimilars effectively treat the condition for which they are prescribed.[21] The following are some of the topics the investigators identified as important for consideration for patient education:

- definition of a biosimilar, including its comparable safety and efficacy
- education on the delivery device and administration (if applicable)
- insurance coverage and out-of-pocket expense
- patient support services, and how clinical trials for biosimilars compare to that of originators.[21]

An interesting aspect of this survey is that investigators identified a desire by patients for information regarding the biosimilar's manufacturer.[21] For example, 28–29% of diagnosed patients stated that the manufacturer's identity was "very influential" in their decision to try a biosimilar.[21] In addition, 10–14% reported that this knowledge was "extremely influential; and 46–48% of diagnosed patients who had participated in support groups felt that the manufacturer identity was "very" or "extremely" influential in their decision.[21] Although it is important to provide all patient-requested education, they should also be informed that a biosimilar from a more well-known manufacturer is not inherently superior to one from a less familiar company. All biosimilars regardless of manufacturer must meet the same FDA-established standards.[2]

Resources

The FDA has posted on its web site information on biosimilars for consumers.[22] This content reviews the basic elements of how biosimilars compare to generics and how they are approved. In addition, the European Commission has also published an information guide for patients, entitled, "What I need to know about Biosimilar Medicines."[23] The guide covers topics similar to the FDA and addresses additional issues such as the roles and responsibilities of the physician, pharmacist, and patient in the use of biosimilars. The document also includes links to other resources from European patient organizations.

WHEN TO EVALUATE

Over the development time frame of a biosimilar, there are currently several milestones:

- the date of the initial approval
- the launch date of a biosimilar, which may be later due to patent litigation issues[24]
- the date of launch of additional biosimilar competition for the same reference product.

When should a biosimilar evaluation take place? As with most issues, there is no one correct answer for every organization. Even though a proactive review would seem desirable, an organization may be resource-constrained and evaluation of a biosimilar, especially for an agent with limited use, may not be appropriate. In organizations with a high degree of use and resource capabilities, a preemptive review prior to final launch would be appropriate.

A review at the time of approval, yet before official launch enables an institution to make a formulary determination and begin preparatory inventory and data management changes necessary to support a conversion. This timeline would enable the pharmacy department to educate all related stakeholders in advance as well as alter purchasing patterns to deplete inventory of the originator.

A Proactive and Global Approach

In addition to preemptive evaluation of biosimilars, some institutions are working with their Pharmacy and Therapeutics Committees to grant pharmacy the discretion to decide whether to remain with an originator or convert to a biosimilar.[25] Rather than conducting a formulary review with each biosimilar approved, pharmacists can establish parameters with their medical staff through which product selection could occur based on a formulary review coupled with an analysis of financial and economic factors. Obviously, not all organizations and/or prescribers will be comfortable with such an approach. Still, some institutions have been successful in educating their physicians on the strength and validity of biosimilar approval as well as obtaining this degree of authority.[25]

KEY POINTS

- Successful implementation and adoption of biosimilars will require a modified approach to formulary review.

- Rather than emphasizing clinical trial review, formulary analysis should focus on operational issues related to ensuring the safe ordering, management, administration, and monitoring of biosimilars along with the financial impact for the organization and patients.

- Education of pharmacists, physicians, other clinicians, and patients will determine the success of biosimilar adoption.

CONCLUSION

Unlike generic medications, it is necessary and preferable to conduct a formulary review of biosimilars before their adoption. The focus of this review differs from that of novel biologics. Pharmacists must understand these differences and ensure their physicians embrace the central tenets of the biosimilar approval process. By definition, biosimilars are highly similar to their originator reference products. Pharmacists must navigate a delicate balance between clinical commonality and look-alike/sound-alike issues that could result in adverse events. Successful adoption of biosimilars requires education and pharmacy must take ownership to ensure that such training is provided to all clinicians and patients.

REFERENCES

1. Rumore MM, Vogenberg FR. Biosimilars: still not quite ready for prime time. *PT.* 2016; 41:366,368-75.

2. Title VII: Improving access to innovative medical therapies. Subtitle A: Biologic Price Competition and Innovation provisions of the Patient Protection and Affordable Care Act (PPACA). www.fda.gov/downloads/Drugs/GuidanceComplianceRegulatoryInformation/ucm216146.pdf (accessed 2 Oct. 2017).

3. Griffith N, McBride A, Stevenson JG, Green L. Formulary selection criteria for biosimilars: considerations for US Health-System Pharmacists. *Hosp Pharm.* 2014; 49:813-25.

4. Lucio SD, Stevenson JG, Hoffman JM. Biosimilars: implications for health-system pharmacists. *Am J Health Syst Pharm.* 2013; 70:2004-2017.

5. Tyler LS, Cole SW, May JR et al. ASHP guidelines on the pharmacy and therapeutics committee and the formulary system. *Am J Health Syst Pharm.* 2008; 65:1272-83.

6. Food and Drug Administration. Guidance for industry. Scientific considerations in demonstrating biosimilarity to a reference product, April 2015. www.fda.gov/downloads/drugs/guidancecomplianceregulatoryinformation/guidances/ucm291128.pdf (accessed 2 Oct. 2017).

7. Food and Drug Administration. Guidance for industry. Nonproprietary naming of biological products. http://www.fda.gov/downloads/drugs/guidances/ucm459987.pdf (accessed 2 Oct. 2017).

8. Food and Drug Administration. Guidance for industry. Clinical pharmacology data to support a demonstration of biosimilarity to a reference product, December 2016. www.fda.gov/downloads/Drugs/GuidanceComplianceRegulatoryInformation/Guidances/UCM397017.pdf (accessed 2 Oct. 2017).

9. Food and Drug Administration. Guidance for industry. Biosimilars: questions and answers regarding implementation of the Biologics Price Competition and Innovation Act of 2009, final guidance, April 2015. www.fda.gov/downloads/drugs/guidancecomplianceregulatoryinformation/guidances/ucm444661.pdf (accessed 2 Oct. 2017).

10. Food and Drug Administration. Guidance for industry, draft guidance. Considerations in demonstrating interchangeability with a reference product. www.fda.gov/downloads/Drugs/GuidanceComplianceRegulatoryInformation/Guidances/UCM537135.pdf (accessed 2 Oct. 2017).

11. Food and Drug Administration. Guidance for industry, draft guidance. Labeling for biosimilar products. www.fda.gov/downloads/drugs/guidancecomplianceregulatoryinformation/guidances/ucm493439.pdf (accessed 2 Oct. 2017).

12. McCamish M, Woollett G. The continuum of comparability extends to biosimilarity: how much is enough and what clinical data are necessary? *Clin Pharmacol Ther.* 2013; 93:315-7.

13. Biosimilars approved in the US. www.gabionline.net/Biosimilars/General/Biosimilars-approved-in-the-US (accessed 2 Oct. 2017).

14. Food and Drug Administration. Guidance for industry, draft guidance. Implementation of the "Deemed to be a License" provision of the Biologics Price Competition and Innovation Act of 2009. www.fda.gov/downloads/drugs/guidancecomplianceregulatoryinformation/guidances/ucm490264.pdf (accessed 2 Oct. 2017).

15. Zarxio (filgrastim-sndz) package insert. Princeton, NJ: Sandoz Inc; 2016 April.

16. Granix (tbo-filgrastim) package insert. North Wales, PA: Teva Pharmaceuticals USA, Inc; 2014 December.

17. Barlas S. Early biosimilars face hurdles to acceptance. *PT.* 2016; 41:362-5.

18. Zelentz AD, Ahmed I, Braud EL et al. NCCN biosimilars white paper: regulatory, scientific, and patient safety perspectives. *J Natl Compr Canc Netw.* 2011; 9(suppl 4):S1-22.

19. Cohen H, Beydoun D, Chien D et al. Awareness, knowledge, and perceptions of biosimilars among specialty physicians. *Adv Ther.* 2016; 33:2160-72.

20. Danese S, Fiorino G, Michetti P. Changes in biosimilar knowledge among European Crohn's Colitis Organization [ECCO] members: an updated survey. *J Crohns Colitis.* 2016; 10:1362-5.

21. Jacobs I, Singh E, Sewell KL et al. Patient attitudes and understanding about biosimilars: an international cross-sectional survey. *Patient Prefer Adherence.* 2016; 10:937-48.

22. FDA. Information for Consumers (Biosimilars). https://www.fda.gov/drugs/developmentapprovalprocess/howdrugsaredevelopedandapproved/approvalapplications/therapeuticbiologicapplications/biosimilars/ucm241718.htm (accessed 2 Oct. 2017).

23. What I need to know about Biosimilar Medicines, Information for patient. European Commission. http://ec.europa.eu/growth/tools-databases/newsroom/cf/itemdetail.cfm?item_id=9072&lang=en (accessed 2 Oct. 2017).

24. Malkin BJ. Biosimilars patent litigation in the EU and the US: a comparative strategic overview. *GaBI Journal* 2015; 4:113-7. http://gabi-journal.net/biosimilars-patent-litigation-in-the-eu-and-the-us-a-comparative-strategic-overview.html (accessed 2 Oct. 2017).

25. Traynor K. Filgrastim becomes biosimilar test case for hospitals. *Am J Health Syst Pharm.* 2016; 73:1805-6.

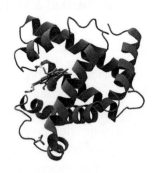

CONCLUSION:
BIOSIMILARS 2023

As introduced in Chapter 9, AbbVie and Amgen recently announced a settlement governing the U.S. launch of adalimumab-atto (Amjevita), a biosimilar of adalimumab (Humira).[1] Under the terms of the agreement, Amgen can begin marketing adalimumab-atto in Europe on October 16, 2018 and in the United States on January 31, 2023. In exchange for this arrangement, Amgen has agreed to dismiss its ongoing patent litigation.[1] Although this agreement does not determine the ultimate disposition of other biosimilar competition such as Boehringer Ingelheim's adalimumab-adbm (Cyltezo), it further reinforces the perspective that AbbVie's patents remain viable beyond 2022. Although the wait for competition is longer than desired, planning toward future events is useful especially for an endeavor as complex as the implementation of the biosimilar paradigm.

Throughout this text, we have discussed the multitude of challenges confronting the biosimilar market including the lack of understanding and continuing evolution of the approval process, uncertainty regarding the role of these agents in clinical practice, ongoing legal disputes, and misaligned and sometimes diametrically opposed value propositions. The number and complexity of barriers could make the return on investment seem questionable. However, if health-system pharmacists commit to the maintenance of a well-informed and consistent focus over the next five years, the extent of value should greatly increase and the difficulty of continued implementation should abate.

2023: THE OPPORTUNITY

By January 1, 2023, the United States will have attained over a decade of experience with the biosimilar concept. This period should also be accompanied by a significant growth in the number of products approved. Biosimilars for filgrastim, infliximab, adalimumab, etanercept, and bevacizumab should ideally be accompanied by licensing for multiple versions of trastuzumab, rituximab, and pegfilgrastim.[2] Again, while the timing of launch of each individual product is subject to multiple variables, more of these molecules will have entered the market. As we have seen in Europe, this degree of familiarity should alter prescriber perceptions and translate into acceptance including the reinforcement provided through expert guideline endorsement.[3,4] In addition, the approval process up to and including interchangeability designations should be established and related guidance information finalized thus mitigating this area of continued uncertainty.

2023: THE CHALLENGE

As mentioned in Chapter 10, the most complicated aspect of the biosimilar experience could be the characterization of an economic and value proposition that supports the consideration of these agents regardless of site of care or payer type. We must continue to monitor actions taken by private payers as well as the government (i.e., Centers for Medicare & Medicaid). As is the case of prescriber familiarity, multiple competitors per originator biologic should also drive additional economic opportunities for biosimilar coverage and use.

THE NEXT WAVE OF BIOSIMILARS

For the above-mentioned reasons as well as greater clinician acceptance and enhanced opportunities for value, the process for future biosimilar adoption should be more straightforward given the very nature of the products approved by 2023. Within the next five years, the U.S. market should have competition for many biologics that define the standard of care for numerous inflammatory and oncology conditions. If the clinical acceptance and a clear financial opportunity can be established for competing versions of infliximab, adalimumab, rituximab, and bevacizumab, the challenge in driving adoption of subsequent agents, such as immunotherapy biosimilars, should be less severe as drugs such as pembrolizumab and nivolumab begin to reach the end of their exclusivities. In biosimilar paradigm, the hard work of analytical characterization paves the way for more focused clinical trial data. Education and reinforcement of the biosimilar methodology today should result in a more efficient and less complicated effort in the future. This degree of acceptance will be essential as our attention will have turned to the advances and associated higher costs of newer immunotherapy products and gene therapies.[5,6]

RESTATING THE OBVIOUS ONE MORE TIME

As mentioned at the beginning of this text, the biosimilar paradigm is a substantial undertaking unto itself. It is also a surrogate example of the work pharmacists must do to establish a correlation between all medications, new or old, small molecule or biologic, generic or biosimilar, and patient outcomes. By improving our comprehension of the regulatory, legal, clinical, financial, and market factors that affect the supply and use of medications, which now include biosimilars, we are better equipped to consider these factors for all other pharmaceuticals we encounter in practice. Success in 2023 and beyond is not just a sustainable market for biologic competition, it is significant progress toward an increasingly stable, more predictable, and truly value-based approach to medication supply and management.

REFERENCES

1.   Sandburg B. Humira biosimilar settlement could be model for other disputes. *The Pink Sheet*, September 28, 2017.

2.   Pending biosimilar applications. The Pink Sheet, FDA Performance Tracker, (subscription) (accessed 4 Oct. 2017).

3.   Danese S, Fiorino G, Michetti P. Changes in biosimilar knowledge among European Crohn's Colitis Organization [ECCO] members: an updated survey. *J Crohns Colitis*. 2016; 10:1362-5.

4.   ECCO position statement on the use of biosimilars for inflammatory bowel disease—an update. *J Crohns Colitis*. 2017; 11:26-34.

5. Lauerman J, Paton J. Novartis' $475,000 price on cancer therapy meets resistance. https://www.bloomberg.com/news/articles/2017-09-22/novartis-s-475-000-price-tag-on-cancer-drug-meets-resistance (accessed 4 Oct. 2017).

6. Check Hayden E. Promising gene therapies pose million-dollar conundrum. *Nature*. 2016; 534:305-6.

INDEX

A

Abatecept, 7

Abbreviated New Drug Application, 12, 73–74

AbbVie, 122, 132, 133, 167

Abciximab, blockbuster, 2

ABP 215, 102, 104, 107

ABP 798, 86

Academy of Managed Care Pharmacy, 122

Adalimumab, 147
    administration of, 133
    adverse reactions to, 115
    biosimilar for, 6, 49, 86
    as blockbuster, 2, 3, 4
    clinically important antibodies to, 118
    expression system for, 23
    IPR and, 132, 133
    manufacturing changes and, 27
    mechanism of action in, 50
    modifications of, 134
    new biosimilars for, 168
    price increases for, 7

Adalimumab-adbm, 86, 121, 167

Adalimumab-atto, 50–51, 86, 121, 133, 161, 167
    clinical studies supporting approval of, 104
    indication coverage for, 100–101, 102
    missing data in, 97

    single switch study of, 109

Adverse events, 123
    biologic, 113–115

Afibercept, 7

Aggregation, 43

Alirocumab, blockbuster, 2

Allergen, 133

America Invents Act, 132

American experience
    approval processes and, 74–75
    biosimilar approvals and, 72–74
    biosimilar guidances and, 76
    generic small molecules, comparable biologics and, 72–75
    interchangeability and, 76–77, 82–83
    mechanisms of action and, 72
    overview of, 71

Amgen, 122, 133, 167

Analytical characterization, statistical approach to, 35–36

Analytical ultracentrifugation, 43

Ariproazole, exclusivity, 5

Assays
    binding, 49
    in vitro biological activity/mechanism of action, 49

Atezolizumab, blockbuster, 2

Atorvastatin
    as blockbuster, 3, 4
    exclusivity and, 5

Average sales price, 144, 145–146

Average wholesale price, 144

B

B1695500, 86
B1695502, 86
Balanced Budget Act of 2018, 148
Bevacizumab
    adverse reactions to, 115
    biosimilar for, 6, 86
    as blockbuster, 3
    expression system for, 23
    manufacturing changes and, 27
    new biosimilars and, 168
    price increase for, 7
Bevacizumab-awwb, 86, 121
    clinical trials for, 107
    indication coverage for, 100–101, 102
    licensure of, 104
Biobetter, 134
Biologic qualifier, 121–122
Biologics
    approvals of, 74
    clinically importance antibodies to, 118
    comparability and, 25–28, 29
    cost of, 4–5
    growth of, 1–2
    recombinant derived, 21
    transition and, 73
Biologics and Biosimilars Collective Intelligence Consortium, 122
Biologics License Applications, 158
Biologics Price Competition and Innovation Act, 5, 12, 161
    approvals and, 72
    aspects of, 73
    biosimilar pathway and, 85
    biosimilar variances and, 122–123
    exclusivity and, 72, 129
    guidance documents and, 76
    interchangeablity and, 80–81
    interchangeability in practice and, 82
    overview of, 71–72
Biosimilarity
    analytical characterization and, 33–34
    analytics and, 33
    clinical data and, 105
    definition of, 71
    goal posts in, 34
    meeting standard of, 49–51
    statistical analytical characterization and, 35–36
Biosimilars, 5–6, 11–18
    analytical characterization and, 51
    approvals of, 15–16
    approved in other countries, 58
    assessing Fab vs. Fc regions in, 49–51
    compared to generics, 15
    compared to originator reference biologic, 35
    definition of, 71
    development milestones for, 163
    Europe's experience with, 15
    exclusivity and, 129
    familiarity with, 16
    high cost of, 13–14
    ligand conjunction and, 44–45
    management infrastructure and, 17
    Medicare reimbursement for, 146–147
    naming, labeling of, 63, 64
    next wave of, 168
    operational differences compared to generics, 16
    perceived drawbacks of, 11–12
    pharmacists support for, 17
    reimbursement (theoretical) for, 145–146
    savings with, 16–17
    in 2023, 167–168
    value checklist for, 149

variability of, 25–26
Biosimilars Forum, 161
Blockbuster drugs, 3–4
    growth of, 4–9
Boehringer-Ingelheim, 122, 167
Brand names, 120
Branded drugs Medicare reimbursement,
    146
Bridging trials, 100–102
British Society of Gastroenterology, 61
British Society of Rheumatology, 62
Brown bagging, 145
Buy and bill model, 145

C

Capillary electrophoresis-sodium dodecyl
    sulfate, 43
Cell expression systems, 22
Certolizumab pegol
    manufacturing changes and, 27
    price increases for, 7
Cetuximab
    amino acid sequence errors and, 41
    expression system for, 23
    manufacturing changes and, 27
    price increases for, 7
Charge heterogeneity, 40
Chinese hamster ovary cells, 22–24
CHS-0214, 86
CHS-1701, 86
Circular dichroism, 41
Clinical data, 105–107, 158
Clinical practice, 102–105, 134
Clinical trials, 91, 127
    bridging trials and, 100–102
    clinical pharmacology data in, 92
    construction of, 109
    equivalence study design in, 95
    extrapolation in, 97–98

FDA's approach to, 91–93
    global, 99–100
    immunogenicity data in, 93, 94
    labeling and, 98–99
    missing data management in, 97
    pharmacodynamics and, 93–94
    pharmacokinetics and, 93–94
    pharmacology studies in action,
        93–95
    scientific considerations in, 92
    superiority vs. equivalence studies in,
        96–97
Clopidogrel
    as blockbuster, 3, 4
    exclusivity and, 5
Comparability, 25–28, 29
Core name, 120
Coverage Gap Discount Program, 147
Creutzfeldt-Jakob disease, 116
Critical quality attributes, 34
CT-P10, 86
Cyclosporine ophthalmic solution, 133

D

Daclizumab, blockbuster, 2
Darbepoetin
    expression system for, 23
    extended dosing and, 134
    price increases for, 7
Data collection, 122–123
Denosumab, 7
Differential scanning calorimetry, 42
Distribution channel selection, 141
Disulfide bonds, 44, 45
Donut hole, 147
Drift, 24
Drug acquisition financial considerations,
    143
Drug Price Competition and Patent Term
    Restoration Act, 11, 127

E

Eculizumab, 7

EP06-101, 94

EP06-103, 94

EP06-105, 94

EP06-109, 94

EP06-302, 94

Epoetin
    European Union and, 59
    pure red cell aplasia and, 116

Epoetin alfa
    adverse reactions to, 115, 116–117
    biosimilar for, 6, 86
    as blockbuster, 2, 3
    immunogenicity and, 118
    price increases for, 7

Epoetin alfa-cgkn, 121

Erythropoietin, 118

Escherichia coli (E coli)
    expression cells, 22–23
    manufacturing success with, 23

Esomeprazole
    as blockbuster, 3
    exclusivity and, 5

Etanercept, 147
    adverse reactions to, 115
    biosimilar for, 6, 49, 86
    as blockbuster, 3, 4
    clinically important antibodies to, 118
    expression system for, 23
    mechanism of action for, 98
    modifications of, 134
    price increases and, 7

Etanercept-szzs, 82, 86, 105, 121, 161
    clinical trials for, 105
    indication coverage for, 100–101, 102

European Crohn's and Colitis Organization, 61, 63, 162

European League Against Rheumatism, 62

European Medicines Agency, 15, 51, 57
    infliximab–dyyb and, 98
    Working Party on Similar Biologic Medicinal Products, 60

European Public Assessment Report, 27

Exclusivity, 78, 127–128
    duration of, 5, 72, 73
    interchangeability and, 80
    new drug applications and, 128
    other and, 128

Expression systems, 22–23

Extrapolation, 63, 64
    clinical trials and, 97–98
    mechanisms of action and, 98
    understanding, 98–99

F

Field flow fractionation, 43

Filgrastim
    biosimilars for, 6, 49, 57–58, 60, 86
    clinical trials for, 104
    expression system for, 23
    global biosimilars for, 57
    mechanism of action for, 98
    United Kingdom's experience with, 59

Filgrastim-bflm, 121

Filgrastim-dyyb, 82–83

Filgrastim-jcwp, 121

Filgrastim-sdnz, 58, 86, 121, 161
    indication coverage for, 100–101, 102
    PK, PD studies and, 93–94
    switching studies for, 107–109

Filgrastim-vkzt, 121

FK238, 86

Food and Drug Administration (FDA), 1
    analytical characterization and similarity assessments by, 52

ANDA and, 12–13

biologic adverse events and, 113–114

biosimilar analytical characterization factors and, 35

biosimilar safety and immunogenicity and, 118–119

biosimilars approved or pending with, 86

biosimilars and originator biologics and, 120–122

BPCI implementations and, 77, 78, 79

clinical pharmacology data and, 78

clinical trials and, 91–93

comparability and, 25–28

core name and, 120

demonstrating biosimilarity and, 51

evaluating analytical similarity and, 80

exclusivity and, 78, 127

extrapolation and, 97–98

formal meetings with, 77

guidance documents of, 76–80

interchangeability and, 79, 81

labeling and, 79

naming biological products and, 78

Orange Book of, 13

Purple Book of, 83–84

quality considerations in biosimilarity and, 77

scientific considerations in biosimilarity and, 77

Sentinel Initiative of, 122

statistical analytical characterization and, 35–36

Formulary management, 14, 153

approval processes for, 158

biosimilar naming, dosage forms and, 153–154

clinical data and, 158

conversion cost and, 159–160

critical document elements and, 154–157

dosage forms differences and, 159

interchangeability and, 160

inventory and, 159

pharmacovigilance and, 160

product naming and, 158

similar biosimilar elements and, 157

Fourier transform infrared spectroscopy, 41, 42

Fructose, 48

Fusion proteins, global biosimilars, 57

G

Generics

acceptance of, 17

annual savings for, 14

experience with, 12–13

initial issues, concerns with, 13

Medicare reimbursement for, 146

model for, 60

prescriptions filled with, 12

Global experience

for biosimilar introductions globally, 57–59

biosimilar position statements on, 61–63

biosimilar success in, 59–60

clinician, physician education, understanding in, 60

developing markets, safety issues in, 66

extrapolation, naming, interchangeability in, 63

financial performance in, 59

interchangeability in, 82–83

Glucagon, expression system for, 23

Glycosylation

impact on pharmacokinetics, pharma-
    codynamics, 48
  PTMs, 44–48
Golimumab
  manufacturing changes and, 27
  price increases for, 7
GP2013, 86
Group purchasing organizations, 142
Growth hormone, clinically important
    antibodies to,118

H

Hatch-Waxman Amendments, 127
Health Canada, 51
  and infliximab–dyyb, 98
Healthcare Common Procedure Coding
    System, 145–146
High pressure liquid chromatography, 40
Higher molecular weight/aggregation, 39
Higher order structure, 38, 41–42
Histidine, 44
Hospitals (inpatient), 143, 144
Hospitals (outpatient), 143, 144
Human insulin, 1
Hydrogen deuterium exchange, 41, 42

I

Immune-mediated reactions, 117–118
Immunogenicity, 113, 115–116, 118
  biosimilars and, 118
  clinical trials and, 93
  focus on, 115–116
Infliximab
  adverse reactions to, 115
  biosimilar for, 6, 49, 60, 63, 86
  as blockbuster, 2, 3, 4
  clinically important antibodies to, 118

expression system for, 23
manufacturing changes and, 27
mechanism of action in, 50
minimally clinically important differ-
    ence, 95
modifications of, 134
new biosimilars for, 168
NOR–SWITCH trial of, 83
price increases for, 7
Infliximab-abda, 86, 121
  clinical studies supporting, 106
  indication coverage for, 100–101, 102
  patent dance and, 131
  single switch study and, 109
Infliximab-dyyb, 49–51, 57–58, 86, 121, 161
  clinical studies supporting approval of,
    103
  extrapolation and, 98
  global studies of, 99–100
  indication coverage for, 100–101, 102
  single switch study for, 109
Information exchange, 130
Insulin, 21
  regular, expression system for, 23
Insulin aspart, 75
Insulin detemir, 75
Insulin glargine
  as blockbuster, 3
  drug approval of, 75
  expression system for, 23
  price increases for, 7
Insulin lispro, 75
Intention to treat, 97
Inter Partes review, 132–133
Interchangeability, 63, 66, 76–77, 79, 86
  BPCI and, 73
  clinical data and, 105–107
  criteria for, 108
  exclusivity and, 80